More than a successful diet progra[...] a complete plan for healthy living [...] need to lose weight *and* gain (or re[...] life. Specifically designed to adapt [...] your lifestyle, it will enable you to achieve and maintain your desired weight and fitness level without giving up the foods you love. Here is a proven system for losing weight and attaining perfect health:

* The Three Keys to Weight Control, Fitness, and Health
* Secrets to Burning Fat and Reshaping Muscle
* How to Heal Your Body with Your Mind
* Healthful and Delicious Low-fat Recipes for Soups, Salads, Main Dishes, and Desserts
* Daily Affirmations and Motivational Techniques to Help You Turn Good Intentions into Action

Find out the secrets of eating the right foods at the right times with the best mind-set for fitness, healing, and health.

STEPHEN TWIGG is one of Britain's most successful holistic health practitioners. He has been an adviser and consultant to well-known figures of British royalty, including the late Princess Diana. During nearly twenty years of private practice, he has numbered among his clientele many celebrities and artists, as well as business and political leaders.

LOVE FOOD...
LOSE WEIGHT

Three Essential Steps to Enjoying Food for Perfect Health

Previously published as
The Kensington Way

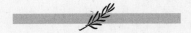

STEPHEN TWIGG

A PLUME BOOK

A Note to the Reader
The ideas, procedures, and suggestions contained in this book are not intended as a substitute
for medical treatment by a physician. The reader should regularly consult a physician in
matters relating to health.

PLUME
Published by the Penguin Group
Penguin Putnam Inc., 375 Hudson Street, New York, New York 10014, U.S.A.
Penguin Books Ltd, 27 Wrights Lane, London W8 5TZ, England
Penguin Books Australia Ltd, Ringwood, Victoria, Australia
Penguin Books Canada Ltd, 10 Alcorn Avenue, Toronto, Ontario, Canada M4V 3B2
Penguin Books (N.Z.) Ltd, 182–190 Wairau Road, Auckland 10, New Zealand

Penguin Books Ltd, Registered Offices: Harmondsworth, Middlesex, England

Originally published by Bantam Books in Great Britain as *The Kensington Diet*.
Previously published in a Dutton edition as *The Kensington Way*.

Published by Plume, a member of Penguin Putnam Inc.

First Plume Printing, January, 2000
10 9 8 7 6 5 4 3 2 1

 REGISTERED TRADEMARK—MARCA REGISTRADA

LIBRARY OF CONGRESS CATALOGING-IN-PUBLICATION DATA

Twigg, Stephen.
    Love food . . . lose weight / Stephen Twigg.
        p.   cm.
    ISBN 0-525-94459-1
        0-452-28152-0 (pbk.)
    1. Reducing diets.   2. Food combining.   3. Nutrition.   I. Title.
    RM222.2.T43   1999
613.2'5—dc21
                                                                98-39945
                                                                CIP

Printed in the United States of America
Set in Transitional 521
Original hardcover design by Leonard Telesca

BOOKS ARE AVAILABLE AT QUANTITY DISCOUNTS WHEN USED TO PROMOTE PRODUCTS OR SERVICES.
FOR INFORMATION PLEASE WRITE TO PREMIUM MARKETING DIVISION, PENGUIN PUTNAM INC.,
375 HUDSON STREET, NEW YORK, NEW YORK 10014.

ACKNOWLEDGMENTS

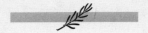

To my family for being there for me

To my friends for their love and support

To my clients for their encouragement and caring

To my teachers, especially Glynn, Stuart, Denise, and Bob, for their wisdom and inspiration

To Peter and Peggy at Alta Vista for their skill, and foresight

Love and thanks to you all—without you, *Love Food . . . Lose Weight* would never have been born

PUBLISHER'S NOTE

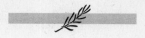

Neither this nor any other book can take the place of individualized medical care or advice. The information in this book is general and not to be considered as professional advice for your specific health problems. If you have a medical condition, are overweight, or are on medication, please talk with your doctor about how dietary changes will affect your health. Sometimes alterations in eating habits can change your need for medication or have other equally important effects. In addition, please consult your doctor before undertaking any substantial increase in your physical activity if you are over forty or suffer from a medical condition. Women who are pregnant or lactating should not consider any weight-reduction diet until they are not pregnant and not lactating, since the health of the woman and her baby relies on both a higher-protein and higher-calorie intake during this time.

The author and the publisher specifically disclaim any responsibility for any liability, loss, or risk, personal or otherwise, which is incurred as a consequence, directly or indirectly, of the use and application of any of the contents of this book.

This book may include words, brand names, and other descriptions of products which are or are asserted to be proprietary names or trademarks. No judgment concerning the legal status of such words is made or implied thereby. Their inclusion does not imply that they have acquired, for legal purposes, a non-proprietary or general significance, or any other judgment concerning their legal status.

CONTENTS

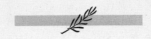

LOVE FOOD...
LOSE WEIGHT

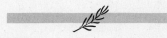

Eat Yourself a Life!

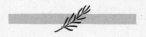

For years my clients have been telling me that I should write a book. Well, here it is—at long, long last!

The reason I felt *Love Food . . . Lose Weight* really had to be written now is because it fills a huge void. With all the books, TV shows, and news articles about food and health, you would think that everything that could possibly be said or written on the subject might have appeared by now. In fact, something vitally important is still missing among all that well-meant advice: *a sensible and practical method for improving your health and controlling your weight.* If that wasn't so, we'd all be getting healthier and slimmer—but we're not.

Despite the fact that we're the most scientifically knowledgeable and medically advanced human beings who have ever lived . . . despite an explosion of popular interest in health, dieting, nutritional supplements, and complementary medicine . . . the harsh reality is we're steadily getting *fatter and sicker.*

You only have to look at the story told by official statistics to realize the truth. In 1972 British government figures showed that one person in every five suffered from some form of chronic, long-standing illness.* Five years later, that figure had risen to one person in every four. Today, it stands at one person in three. If this remorseless trend

*General Household Survey, Office of Population Censuses and Surveys, 1993, HMSO.

continues, pretty soon half the population will be afflicted with one long-term illness or another, if not disability or infirmity. The figures for children, by the way, are even more alarming—in 1972, just eight percent of children suffered from chronic disease, but by 1993, 19 percent were afflicted. Statistics that describe the alarming increase in numbers of clinically obese in the United States tell a similar story. These are grim figures indeed, and I can't understand why they don't provoke more widespread public concern and media interest.

At the same time the average human lifespan is gradually increasing, the general level of health is actually declining. Paradoxically, it seems we have longer to do the things that will eventually cause us to become ill and overweight. In other words, we've found out how to keep ourselves alive longer—so that we can suffer more! For decades governments and medical authorities have poured resources into the treatment—or containment—of ill health, and have all but abandoned the far more important issue of how to *stop* people becoming ill—or overweight—in the first place. One of the consequences of this kind of policy is we haven't really been shown how to stay healthy and slim. Another is today's crippling pressure on our medical facilities, as they falter under the sheer number of ill people requiring a doctor's help. The confusion of private medical insurance schemes available makes sense only when you understand the real problem is people *haven't been taught how to stay well.*

However, this book isn't concerned with statistics (actually, it's more concerned with preventing you from becoming one!). For nearly twenty years I've spent every day of my working life helping some of the world's most wealthy, famous, and powerful people look after their health and appearance. From that particularly privileged and unique viewpoint I've made it my business to learn just what affects our bodies and how we can help them to be healthier and look better. My knowledge comes from being a hands-on body worker. I work physically with my clients' skin, fat, sinews, muscles, and joints. As a therapist, working my clients' bodies every week, sometimes two or three times weekly, over many years I've felt, with my two hands, what their bodies are experiencing. I know—firsthand, as it were—the effects of their diets, their lifestyles, their exercising or lack of it, and even of the way they are feeling about themselves and their lives. By direct touch and frank conversation, I have come to understand what affects people's bodies over a prolonged period of time. This book contains the most important lessons I've learned and truths I've discovered—practical information whose sole purpose is to help you achieve a higher degree of lasting health and happiness than you've ever experienced before.

YES, IT REALLY CAN BE YOU!

How would you like to win the lottery?

You don't need to tell me the answer! If we're honest, most of us would admit that, from time to time, we have fantasies of being enormously wealthy (and, by the way, even millionaires dream of being billionaires!). In our society, money buys freedom—freedom from the worry of debt, freedom from the daily nine-to-five grind, freedom to enjoy the kind of lifestyle your heart desires. Well, imagine winning the lottery and becoming as rich as you could ever want. What difference do you think it would make to your health or to your shape? Would you suddenly have the key to a healthier, fitter, and more attractive body? Perhaps you think the wealthy are naturally more sporty and athletic and into fitness regimes? Not so, I'm afraid. There are just as many couch potatoes among the rich as there are among the rest of us!

Immense wealth wouldn't make a great deal of difference to your health or your size and shape. Everything I've observed from two decades of experience with the great and the good of this world testifies that wealth, and the fame that often goes with it, is a greater rather than a lesser burden on health and appearance. Most of my clients have become my friends over the years we've worked together. They've shared their thoughts and feelings, hopes and dreams with me—so I know all too well how some people become overburdened with the sadness and pain of a life distorted by fame and great wealth.

Now, it's true that money can be very useful for repairing your health or appearance *after* they've been ravaged by the many things in modern life that can affect them. Nothing I have ever seen or heard, though, has convinced me that money can buy true health or a perfectly shaped body. The idea that you can somehow buy a perfect shape, or that you can be fully well without making some sort of effort yourself, is a false dream. If you want to keep or improve your health, if you want to look better or stay in good shape, *you* have to *do* something, and the sooner you start the better. That's an inescapable truth, and because it is so, you are in exactly the same position as the wealthiest people in the world.

And there, you may think, lies another problem. Don't you have to really work at looking good? Don't you have to spend, if not money, a lot of time and effort? Doesn't it become a real struggle to do all the things you have to do to take care of yourself?

The answer is: No! In most cases a close companion to wealth is a lifestyle which imposes immense demands. In the face of those demands I've seen many struggle with health problems or despair about the way they look—and don't forget, for some their looks are among their most important assets. Great wealth and high position often bring immense stresses, unique pressures, much anxiety, and always—*always*—a chronic shortage of time. Can you imagine what it's like to be constantly in debt to the second hand of the clock? To have a hundred and one people constantly clamoring to devour every precious minute of your life? Many of my wealthiest clients probably have *less* time than you to spend on themselves.

Part of my success with my clients—and one of the key reasons why *Love Food . . . Lose Weight* is going to work for you—is that I've been able to show them how they can make a real difference by changing *very little* about their everyday lives. In other words, it doesn't take as much time as they thought, it doesn't take as much effort, and above all, they *don't* have to give up as many of the good things in life as they feared. After all, if you are accustomed to eating the best food money can buy in the nicest restaurants, you are hardly eager to give up that luxury and seek out lentils, or bean sprouts, or any other food you don't really like—no matter how often you're told it is good for you!

When I say "make a difference," I'm talking about changes they might never have expected or even imagined possible. I mean differences to their level of *general health* and their ability to stay healthier *longer* and *more easily*. I mean differences to their appearance, in their weight, shape, skin, and muscle tone. That also means a difference to the way they move: their general presence, their self-image, and self-esteem. That means a difference to the way they feel about life and how they deal with it. I've been able to show them that far from being a burden, making such changes can be easy, enjoyable, and exciting!

That's the beauty of understanding what really affects your health. If you know how to help your body get the best from everything you eat, then you can enjoy any food. If you know how best to spend your time caring for yourself, then you need to spend very little to get the results you want. If you know how the human body really responds to exercise, you'll find you won't have to do very much to get the benefits you are aiming for.

My job is to know those things and to help people make them a normal part of their lives. *Love Food . . . Lose Weight* is all about making a difference—it's a system that works for the most demanding, time-starved, and discerning people in the world—people who are the least likely to accept difficult or time-consuming changes to their lifestyles. And if it works for them, then I promise you—we're going to make it work for you, too!

ORIGIN OF THE *LOVE FOOD . . . LOSE WEIGHT* DIET

It came as quite a shock when, early in my career, I discovered that I didn't have all the answers I needed.

I spent many years of learning physical techniques of massage and manipulation which I hoped would enable me to alleviate all kinds of problems. But as I became more experienced and worked with different teachers and different methods, I realized that physical therapy, while being a wonderful system for helping others, did not have the answers to all their problems. Apparently straightforward muscle or joint problems would respond well to treatment, but then inexplicably recur. Some problems would not respond at all for long periods of time, and then suddenly disappear. I wanted to find out the reason for these peculiar reactions.

Clearly the physical, mechanical systems of the body I was concerned with were being influenced by something other than simple mechanical forces. But what else could cause acute or chronic muscle and joint pain? What could disrupt normal tissue tone so rapidly or make muscles so completely unresponsive to exercise? I had to discover this "hidden factor" if I was going to be able to offer effective solutions to my clients' problems.

My quest was given added urgency when I began to suffer some health problems of my own. Clients often assume that their therapists are somehow superhuman and miraculously immune to the afflictions of lesser mortals. Well, this one certainly wasn't! I had always suffered badly from migraines, but now the attacks became depressingly regular and so excruciating that they immobilized me for days at a time—forcing me to cancel appointments and imprisoning me in a darkened room until they finally passed. Even worse, I found I was mysteriously putting on weight, becoming bloated after meals and feeling increasing discomfort in many of my joints. Giving physical therapy can be a real strain on a therapist if his or her body isn't in good shape. I found that the tendons of my hands were very susceptible to strain and inflammation, my legs ached and, strangely, my eyes were extremely sensitive to bright light.

It was then I made one of the most important discoveries of my life about the way I was eating. I had been causing my own problems all along with bad food combinations. Food combining came into my life apparently by accident, but at exactly the right moment— when I needed it the most. In a similar way, I hope this book has also come into *your* life at just the right moment, when you are in a position to really benefit from it. You know, there really is no such thing as coincidence.

My childhood was spent in the relatively austere fifties and early sixties. Fish sticks and burgers and french fries had just been launched onto the mass market. Our family's meals were based on value for money and what could be cooked quickly and easily for four children by a working mother. "Healthy eating" simply wasn't something we considered.

Later, my twenties and thirties coincided with the boom in convenience meals and foods imported from around the world. Although dieting and health foods were rapidly becoming more common, my own basic eating pattern didn't change substantially—the main one being the replacement of french fries and burgers with rice and chicken curry, or pasta with Bolognese sauce.

Then my health crisis struck. My general level of health and physical shape was slowly but clearly deteriorating. I put a lot of effort into eating what was supposed to be healthy food bought expensively at health food shops. Brown rice and whole wheat pasta took the places of their refined counterparts in my meals—to little positive effect.

When I was told about food combining, I had never even considered that there might be a different way of eating than the bad combinations I was used to. I had never heard of another way of mixing foods in meals, despite the fact it has been widely known and respected as a healthy eating system in Europe for decades. I was skeptical, but by then I had become desperate enough to try anything.

I have to be candid and tell you that food combining was initially very difficult for me. The program I undertook was a time-consuming, highly detailed scheme requiring considerable discipline and organization. The program was designed for the totally committed and assumed total commitment for the three months it lasted. I literally had to change my whole life pattern in order to follow the required procedures. I was extremely lucky to be in a position that I could find the time needed to acquire and cook the special foods I ate, and overcome the reactions I suffered to some of the processes that were used.

Nevertheless, I persevered—and it worked. While I benefited hugely in many ways from that old-style food-combining program, I knew not a single one of my clients would be prepared to follow a similar regime. They simply didn't have the time to have their lives so disrupted by what was required, regardless of the improvements they would have achieved.

In short, there was no way I could use the new insights and knowledge I had gained for the benefit of my clients.

WHAT'S REALLY GREAT ABOUT FOOD COMBINING?

Food combining is the greatest diet system in existence, but it doesn't always make sense. It's been around since even before its best-known proponent, Dr. William Howard Hay, championed its use by the medical profession in the early twentieth century. Since then it has helped countless people recover their health and bring their weight under control permanently.

Food combining, or the art of compatible eating, attracts some disbelief because superficially it doesn't seem to make sense. The main rule—don't allow protein-rich foods to be in your stomach with starch- or sugar-rich foods—seems to be nonsense when you think that people in all cultures have been doing just that for centuries. How can this combination be so bad for you?

People have been combining their foods the ways they do more for historical and social reasons than for nutrition, and just because people have been doing something for centuries doesn't prove that it's good for you! I like to use the analogy of the air we breathe to demonstrate what I mean when I answer this most obvious of objections to food combining.

We know the air we breathe is often tainted by car exhaust and industrial fumes. At times we can actually taste or smell the pollution as we breathe it in. Sometimes we're not aware of it in the air, but we still know it's there. We don't, however, drop dead by the side of the road as we breathe it—our bodies try to cope. Year after year lung disease and asthma increase; breathing difficulties affect millions now, and still we cope—because we have to. Some of us even adapt to it a little, becoming townies who don't notice what a countryside dweller would feel immediately. However, this doesn't mean we wouldn't be *a lot healthier* if we managed to remove the pollution from our air.

It's the same with food combining. Yes, you can get by eating poorly combined food. Your long-suffering but wonderfully durable body will adapt and try to cope with almost any kind of mistreatment, but damage is gradually being done. Just because you can get by doesn't mean you *should*—if you are sensible. With the air you breathe, you have no choice. With the food you eat, you *do* have a choice, at every meal. The choice is whether to get healthier and slimmer and *more alive* . . . or not.

Poor food combining and certain other common eating habits result in increased amounts of toxins in the body. Toxins are internal pollutants that prevent your body working as efficiently as it wants to. Toxins directly damage your system, and cause your body to divert vital energy and essential biochemical resources to deal with the damage they inflict.

The fact is, different types of food are digested best in different chemical environments, sometimes in different parts of your digestive system. Put the two main food types, proteins and carbohydrates, together in a meal and neither is digested particularly well, and *that* increases the toxicity your body has to deal with. That results in increasing levels of discomfort and harm as your body is forced to do its best with what you're giving it every day. But when you eat food that is well combined, your body is not put under the stress of having to deal with foods it can't digest easily, or their toxic end products.

Love Food . . . Lose Weight shows you how to use simple yet powerful techniques to help you reverse the problems poor food combinations cause. When you combine food successfully, your body benefits from better nutrition with less effort and has resources and energy to spare to remove existing toxins and *heal itself.*

Properly combining your food—as explained in this book—can achieve terrific results for you, including making you look and feel healthier, happier, younger, and more zestful. However, in all honesty I have to tell you that, by itself, food combining doesn't have *all* the answers. Other bad eating habits besides poor combining have equally damaging effects on your body. And factors other than food cause us to *use* food badly. That's why *Love Food . . . Lose Weight* is unique—it's a complete system, which is *based* upon food combining but not *limited* to food combining. In effect, *Love Food . . . Lose Weight* transforms an already powerful eating system into a truly amazing one!

Love Food . . . Lose Weight is an approach to diet for the new millennium. It not only combines food well in more delicious ways than you can imagine, but combines the best and most effective methods for making food work for your health into a wonderful method of self-care. Nor is *Love Food . . . Lose Weight* a rigid, exclusive system. Most other diet and health strategies you've heard of can be used alongside it. In fact, when used with *Love Food . . . Lose Weight*, most other approaches to health and slimming work even better.

In the years since first discovering food combining, I've transformed my own health. I've investigated food combining and other diet systems, and I've studied and validated many other methods of improving the health, shape, and vitality of the body. I've also explored methods of self-care and self-improvement from fields as diverse as exercise, psychology, alternative medicine, metaphysics, and ancient philosophies. Up to now my methods have been used exclusively for my clients. Now I'm going to share them with you as well. You can learn the secrets of how to make food your best friend in your efforts to be healthy, vital, and slim for life.

WHY THE *LOVE FOOD . . . LOSE WEIGHT* DIET WILL SUCCEED FOR YOU!

Most diets and systems of health care and weight control adopt a more or less scientific approach to bring about improvements. Their methods are based on one simple premise: each problem has an identifiable cause, and all that's required to solve the problem is to address that cause.

This viewpoint is narrow, blinkered, and obviously wrong—yet widely accepted. It suggests that excess weight, for example, can be controlled simply by finding the right diet or the correct exercise or even the right drug. So you'll find low-fat diets, calorie-controlled diets, calorie-rotation diets, low-salt diets, low-sugar diets, high-protein diets, and detoxifying diets. There are exercise programs ranging from aerobics to yoga and drugs or herbs to speed up your metabolism, purge water from your body, or stop fat from sticking to it. The picture is similar with solutions to health problems.

The idea of simple solutions to simple problems is seductive. The concept fits nicely with the scientific notion of your body as a machine that can be repaired when you find the part that's broken, but it doesn't fit with the *reality* of what living things are and how they work.

We know that illnesses don't affect everyone the same way. They strike different people at different rates or maybe not at all. The same is true with excess weight. Some people become huge while eating very little, while others are rake-thin even though they eat enormous amounts. When we look at the broader picture, instead of searching among the minute details of human chemical and organic mechanisms, we find that health relies on many diverse elements. Illness and weight problems develop from a coincidence of many factors, not from just a single cause. Food, environment, social and family issues, mental attitude and emotional state, activities, behavior, and genetic makeup all play a part. Together they create a pattern of underlying health that develops, shifts and changes, and from time to time produces the conditions from which your health and weight problems arise. No one can say to what degree each factor plays a role for any particular person in any particular problem. Such is the way of living things.

No wonder we prefer to accept the simpler picture of "one solution for one problem" painted by science. Inherent in that approach, though, is a serious drawback: the solution to one difficulty can be the forerunner of another problem. Methods for health and shape improvement aimed at only *one* factor among many can work quite well for a while. But these methods don't actually achieve much in the long term, and frequently they can cause more harm than good. By aggressively altering just one component, such as diet, for instance, other factors essential to health and well-being can be disturbed, eventually causing the same problem to recur or another, worse problem to arise in its place.

The main reason *Love Food . . . Lose Weight* is so successful is that *it works at many levels* and simultaneously affects all the elements that play a role in your health and well-being. While it works to improve your overall health for the long term, it also helps with any problems that have already occurred. It even uses methods to help inhibit problems that are in the process of arising before you even know they are there.

Let me explain by telling you about one of my clients—Margaret.* She was fifty-five when we were first introduced, as usual, by another client. Her problems came in droves. During the twelve years prior to our meeting she had endured surgery for cancer of the bowel and a further two operations for the adhesions caused by the original surgery. Adhesions result when internal surgical scars heal and the scar material becomes attached to adjacent organs or tissue. As you can well imagine, this can be very painful and cause serious problems if, as in Margaret's case, it involves an organ like the bowel, which works by strong, even violent, muscular contractions along its length to expel waste material. Margaret had frequent discomfort and constant anxiety about the possibility of her bowel requiring further surgery. Surgeons had told her they were extremely concerned about the outcome if any further operations for adhesions were needed.

*The name and other details have been changed to protect the privacy of the individual concerned.

But that was by no means the end of Margaret's troubles. She also bore the all-too-visible scars of open-heart bypass surgery—those elongated "zips" both in the leg where surgeons remove a healthy blood vessel and all along her sternum where the vessel is inserted as new plumbing around the heart. And, just for good measure, she was quite overweight and suffered from persistent muscular problems in her neck, shoulders, back, and legs.

Margaret and I got down to business. While I physically worked on her aches and pains, she set about learning the principles of *Love Food . . . Lose Weight*. Five years later, her diet had changed dramatically. She became a convert and found out that if she stepped too far beyond the good eating rules outlined in this book, her problems would start to return. She combined food according to *Love Food . . . Lose Weight* principles most of the time, she learned which foods affected her badly and avoided them, and she rotated those foods that might have become a problem. She discovered that water is a panacea for many of her problems and learned how to use it to prevent or respond to minor symptoms of discomfort. Margaret's general health improved greatly. Among the many symptoms that were effectively controlled was the abdominal discomfort she had learned to dread. When Margaret had to have more surgery for another long-standing problem, doctors and surgeons were amazed at her recovery, which was rapid and far beyond their expectations. Five years after her first appointment with me, Margaret had more energy than ever before, understood what she could and could not do with her diet, understood the needs of her own body, and thus was able to care for her own health. She succeeded in losing weight and maintained an active social life in which dining with friends played a major role.

Then one day her doctors told her she needed an emergency operation.

It happened like this. She returned to London after a weekend country house party, and suddenly began to suffer severe abdominal pains. Quickly, she went to her doctor, highly apprehensive about a possible return of the adhesion problems. "This is an emergency, and we need to get you to a specialist—now" was the doctor's instant diagnosis, and he personally took her—straight away. A half hour examination and a complete review of her history led both doctor and specialist to advise immediate surgery, despite the very real risk. Dismayed by this, and in no state to make a clear-headed decision, Margaret faced a truly dreadful dilemma. Should she consent to immediate surgery, with the severe risk it entailed, or should she refuse—and continue to endure agonizing pain?

Luckily, Margaret retained enough presence of mind to ask about something neither the doctor nor specialist had mentioned in their inquiries.

"Could anything I've recently eaten," she asked, "be responsible for what's happening to me?"

Maybe, answered the doctors. So then and there, in great pain but desperate to avoid an emergency operation, Margaret tried to remember everything she'd eaten over the past seventy-two hours.

That's what saved Margaret from going under the surgeon's knife again, with possibly grave consequences. Although her doctors had never previously told her that certain foods, particularly certain fruits, might cause her already sensitive bowel to overwork, she had learned, from *Love Food . . . Lose Weight*, how foods could affect her body. My frequent inquiries about her diet and its effects on her were what she recalled, luckily, in the specialist's consulting room. Before returning to London from her weekend away, Margaret had enjoyed several of her favorite fruits: four ripe and delicious fresh plums, complete with their soft skins. Those plums were the cause of her acute pains.

Margaret resolved her own difficulty without surgery, by drinking several extra glasses of water every day for a week. Today, this remarkable lady enjoys a new sense of self-assurance and calm which permeates her life in many other ways. Not only is she more confident about her health and her ability to look after it, but she is also more assertive with her medical advisers, less liable to be bothered by minor problems for which she has a range of responses from her *Love Food . . . Lose Weight* experiences, and more relaxed generally. Margaret's story shows not only that these diet principles can improve health, but that they can make real differences on *many* levels. Someone who has been shown *how to stay well* can actively assume responsibility for their own health—with clearly beneficial consequences.

Love Food . . . Lose Weight, in contrast to most other diets, is a powerful, multifaceted approach for the multidimensional situation that produces your health and shape. It deals not with cause and effect in isolation, but with how you function as a whole person—not just as a body-machine of organs, glands, bones, and chemistry.

If all that seems rather daunting, please don't worry! The most remarkable thing about the *Love Food . . . Lose Weight* diet is how very *easy* it is. When you enhance the natural ways you function, guiding yourself to your goal rather than trying to force yourself to become how you want to be, you'll engage a quite remarkable spontaneous process which will help you—as you will soon see.

WHAT YOU CAN EXPECT
FROM THE *LOVE FOOD . . . LOSE WEIGHT* DIET

You'll start with what seems like a real drawback but which rapidly becomes a revelation. Changing the way you combine your food can appear daunting, but with the *Love Food . . . Lose Weight* way it becomes a *pleasure*.

No diet or health system in the world will demand or even deserve your wholehearted involvement if you don't enjoy it. You're going to discover that food that's good to eat can be good for you—when you know how to eat it.

We live in an age when food culture is a major part of our pleasure in life. International and haute cuisine are featured daily on television and in the media. Foods from around the world are readily available in every supermarket. Our homes are becoming gastronomic testing grounds, and scores of wonderful restaurants tempt us with new and more wonderful food creations all the time. One of the great breakthroughs with *Love Food . . . Lose Weight* is recognizing that, for the average person trying to make improvements to their health and weight, it simply isn't necessary to dramatically alter what you want to eat.

> As long as you know how to eat correctly, you can eat anything you like! In fact, there are some very compelling reasons why you should continue to eat what you want, which you'll discover soon.

So when you ask what you have to give up to be healthy, slim, and full of zest for life, I can honestly reply *nothing*! The real beauty of this diet is in the food. If you don't believe me, just look at the recipes and you'll see what I mean!

Of course, we don't always have the time to cook wonderful meals. The modern lifestyle presents challenges to anyone who wants to take care of their health and weight. The beauty of the *Love Food . . . Lose Weight* is its flexibility. It's a totally *realistic* method that lends itself to any lifestyle and whatever aspirations you have for yourself. At its simplest it is a *practical* way of restoring your general health. Just use the basic diet and over time, with minimum effort and without depriving yourself of what you like, you'll feel better and more alive day by day. At its most powerful, *Love Food . . . Lose Weight* is a vehicle for amazing self-transformations that will affect every area of your life.

Another important aspect of *Love Food . . . Lose Weight* is that it works to motivate your good *intentions* into worthwhile *actions*. The road to hell, they say, is paved with good intentions. All the good intentions in the world won't make anything happen on their own.

The key to motivation is to know how your mind works. The reason most diets and health programs fail is that they do not take into account the fact that your mind often acts to *hinder* what you are trying to achieve—or that it can be taught to *help* you instead. Virtually all change is resisted at some stage, and unless you know how to approach change skillfully you are not likely to succeed, regardless of the benefits a diet could bring you.

When you use the *Love Food . . . Lose Weight*, you'll learn that how you *think* about yourself affects every part of your body and mind, and that what you *eat* can affect the ways you think about yourself! You'll learn that there is a way of changing your diet that will help you think more positively and powerfully, and that some changes to what you eat can make you feel disabled and lacking in confidence to the point of giving up on any diet.

I'll show you how to identify negative thoughts and feelings and switch them around until they become a *positive help* toward achieving what you want.

It's said that nothing succeeds like success, and that gives us an insight into the unique reason for the success of the *Love Food . . . Lose Weight*. The combination of diet and supporting methods you're going to be using leads, after a while, to an interesting phenomenon. The *more* you use this diet, the *less* you'll feel like returning to the ways you ate before. You'll begin to experience *spontaneous change*.

You'll find yourself automatically choosing healthier eating options. Your tastes will change away from processed foods, high-salt or -sugar foods, and poor combinations. You just won't like them as much as before. You'll find yourself eating less without thinking about it, and you'll find your food cravings have greatly diminished.

How does this happen? When you engage your body and mind together in improving your diet, you'll discover you have a natural tendency to prefer the healthiest ways of doing things and can easily let go of old ways that no longer help you. When you eat in ways that make you feel and function well, you'll find any tendency to slide back into bad old habits blocked by preferences for what's good for you. It's a wonderful feeling to realize you are quite spontaneously choosing to eat what's best for you and that you're enjoying it more than the old diet you used to eat. It is the greatest *positive reinforcement* of all— you just find yourself forgetting to eat badly!

It's part of human nature not to embark on any new endeavor you are presented with, unless it's accompanied by *information* that persuades you it's safe and worth trying. Throughout *Love Food . . . Lose Weight,* you'll find the information you need to enable you to take each step easily and naturally. The information isn't presented in the form of dry, dusty data drawn from science journals, however. Rather, it's an accumulation of evidence and arguments that your own innate common sense will tell you is right.

What you're going to learn will be further strengthened by the greatest authority of all: *your own experience.* The information you'll get from *Love Food . . . Lose Weight* will be verified as you use it to become healthier and slimmer. You'll gain insight into the most fascinating subject of all—*yourself*—until you understand yourself and what is best for you so well, you'll be able to maintain your health as long as you want.

Ultimately, the most profound insight you'll gain from using *Love Food . . . Lose Weight* is the realization of your own uniqueness. Yes, we're all similar—but not the *same.* You'll appreciate how different you are from any other person on the planet, and how you became that way. Because you are absolutely unique and extraordinarily special, you'll discover the solutions to your problems have to be different from anyone else's. With *Love Food . . . Lose Weight*, you'll find out what your own unique solutions really are.

So now, let's begin to discover *your* solutions!

CHAPTER

2

Your Food—Friend or Foe?

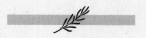

We eat food in the expectation that it will keep us alive and well—but the food you eat can become the most serious threat to your health and well-being that you'll ever have to face. I'm going to describe for you the strange twist of circumstances that turns your food from your best friend into a dreadful foe.

This threat is not from occasional contamination by bacteria or from adulteration with chemicals and additives, serious though these sometimes are. The threat isn't even from particular foods like fats or sugar or salt, which most of us realize by now can eventually become harmful. The most serious threat comes from ordinary, unremarkable foods you eat all the time.

Without being aware of it you may be choosing foods, every day, that are shortening your life, making you ill, disrupting your weight and shape, and preventing you from being as happy, contented, and successful as you could be.

The foods you routinely choose to eat can be creating a *deteriorating situation* in your mind and body which becomes more and more difficult to correct as time goes by. The very problems you perhaps blame on aging may actually be the accumulating effects of your poor eating.

Every day, day in day out, you may be making the biggest mistakes of your life—because you aren't really sure what bad eating is.

YOUR DIET—WHAT'S REALLY GOING WRONG?

We all have some ideas about what bad eating is, don't we?

We're told often enough and in no uncertain terms about too much fat, too much salt, too much sugar, not enough fruit or vegetables, too many additives, too many refined foods, animal products, non-organically produced foods . . . the list seems endless. No wonder many people just throw their hands up in despair and shout, "So what *is it* OK to eat?"

Most of this type of advice about bad eating is typical of the "body as machine" approach to health that's so dominant today. The fact that it often flies in the face of our instincts and experience is what makes it so confusing.

Let me explain. Not so long ago in Britain, the government tried to define the quantities of different types of foods we should all eat daily in order to be healthy. Now, most of us realize we ought to eat a wide range of foods for the energy and nutrients we need. Many of us also have some idea that everyone needs the full spectrum of vitamins, minerals, amino acids, and trace elements available from food. But do we all need exactly the same amounts of each nutrient? Do we all need exactly the same proportions of each food with the same frequency?

Think about it for a moment—does a weightlifter need the same diet as a long-distance runner? No, of course not. If they both ate the same diet, one of them at least is going to have problems in their chosen sport. Activity and physique influence what you need to eat.

Does a 350-pound wrestler need the same diet as a 150-pound computer programmer? Of course he doesn't, and if they both ate the same diet, one of them is not going to be able to do his job properly for long. People who have a mainly sedentary lifestyle or who use more mental than physical energy have different requirements from their food.

Do men need the same diet as women? Now, there's a question! Of course, it depends on the man and woman, but if you live with anyone of the opposite gender, you probably know you both choose completely different foods when you are eating separately. Even gender influences what you choose to eat.

Think of someone you know who always seems angry or tense—

now think of someone who is placid and calm. Do they both eat the same foods in the same amounts? Not likely, is it—because personality and mental attitude also influence what you need from food.

Obvious examples like these help to illustrate that across the spectrum of human form, activity, temperament, and personality, we each have different needs from food.

Also, consider this—what if all the characters I've mentioned did take the advice they were given and ate exactly the same amounts of the same foods? Do you think they would each enjoy the same benefits from what they consumed?

No, of course they wouldn't. Even if everything else was equal, digestion is not. People's digestive systems may be based on the same model, but they vary quite a lot and they don't work the same either.

Just as faces and bodies are externally different in shape, size, and function, so are internal organs. Your organs of digestion differ in size, shape, and effectiveness from everyone else's. Your stomach acid can be different, your gall bladder and liver function may vary, and your bowel activity isn't necessarily the same.

Not only are there these inherent differences, but the passage of time, lifestyle, and diet can gradually alter the efficiency of any particular organ or of an entire digestive system—but in different ways and at different rates for different people.

ONE PERSON'S POISON . . .

My point here is to emphasize something you instinctively know already, namely, your needs from food are *completely unique*. What you need from food is different from anyone else. What your body does with food when it passes through your system is different from what another person's will do when they eat identical food.

Assessing individual foods, or types of food, then defining them as bad or good for health or weight control can be very misleading. When you take into account how diverse we all are, and how dissimilar are our needs and uses of food, giving the same advice to everyone, as if we were all identical, is nonsense.

To start looking for what's wrong with your eating solely in a list of good and bad foods will not help you very much at all, because you don't know if the evidence which leads to that distinction is true for you. Even if the evidence is valid, you might ask, "How valid for me?" A food that influences one person's health or shape significantly may have only a marginal effect on another.

Furthermore, you are most probably being affected by many suspect foods, all at the same time. The combinations and quantities of foods you're using are unique to you. With all these variables you can't know which food, if any, is really affecting you seriously or in what circumstances it's doing so.

Many diet experts are worried by the trend that argues some foods as entirely bad for everyone. They are concerned about the ways many people, through lack of sufficient knowledge and understanding, respond by completely rejecting foods that may be very important to them.

The whole idea of being able to analyze your diet, cut out one or two foods, and then include one or two others to somehow create a major benefit to your health doesn't hold water. Similarly, the notion you can adjust your intake of a few key foods to alter your shape or size substantially and permanently is not practical, not effective, and not very valid. One person's food can indeed be another's poison.

Plenty of people tell you what you shouldn't eat and why, but no one seems to be able to tell you why you eat what's bad for you in the first place or how you can stop—until now.

There's a similar problem with advice about how much it's OK to eat.

It's true that in our modern and developed society most people are eating more than they need to. The question it would be most useful to have the answer to is not, How much should you be eating? but, Why do you eat too much in the first place? More precisely still, How can you stop eating more than you need?

Just for a moment glance over the list that follows. I've collected it from my own personal experiences, from the experiences of my clients, and from reports about the effects of food combining from elsewhere. All the health problems and conditions mentioned here have substantially improved or been completely resolved when the people suffering them used better food combining.

- ❏ Abdominal distension
- ❏ Acne
- ❏ Allergies
- ❏ Anal itching/hemorrhoids
- ❏ Arthritis
- ❏ Asthma
- ❏ Bags under eyes
- ❏ Bloating
- ❏ Blood pressure
- ❏ Body odor
- ❏ Burping
- ❏ Cellulite
- ❏ Cholesterol
- ❏ Clarity of thought, lacking
- ❏ Cold extremities
- ❏ Cold sores
- ❏ Cold sweats
- ❏ Colon health
- ❏ Complexion problems
- ❏ Confidence problems
- ❏ Dark circles under eyes
- ❏ Duodenal ulcer
- ❏ Eczema
- ❏ Eyes sensitive to light
- ❏ Fatigue
- ❏ Fingernail problems
- ❏ Flatulence
- ❏ Fluid retention
- ❏ Food cravings
- ❏ Food intolerance
- ❏ Frequent colds
- ❏ Gallbladder problems
- ❏ Hair condition problems
- ❏ Hay fever
- ❏ Headaches
- ❏ Hunger pangs
- ❏ Hyperactivity
- ❏ Hyperglycemia
- ❏ Hypoglycemia
- ❏ Indigestion
- ❏ Insomnia
- ❏ Irritability
- ❏ Joint pain
- ❏ Joint swelling
- ❏ Lack of appetite
- ❏ Lack of energy
- ❏ Libido problems
- ❏ Low back pain
- ❏ Melancholy/depression
- ❏ Migraine
- ❏ Mood swings
- ❏ Mouth ulcers
- ❏ Muscle aches
- ❏ Muscle cramps
- ❏ Muscle tension
- ❏ Muscle tone problems
- ❏ Nausea
- ❏ Neck and shoulder pain
- ❏ Nervousness
- ❏ Pallor
- ❏ Peptic ulcer
- ❏ Persistent thirst
- ❏ PMS
- ❏ Psoriasis
- ❏ Psychological disorders
- ❏ Puffy eyes
- ❏ Self-esteem problems
- ❏ Sensitivity to cold
- ❏ Sinus conditions
- ❏ Size changes
- ❏ Skin quality problems
- ❏ Sleep problems
- ❏ Stress
- ❏ Temperament problems
- ❏ Tinnitus
- ❏ Weight gain
- ❏ Weight loss
- ❏ Yeast imbalance

How many can you tick off for yourself or someone you know?

This catalogue of ills indicates that the way you combine your food is in some way affecting just about every part and function of your body and mind. The list covers all types of problems, from minor ailments to major diseases, from body dysfunction to personality difficulties and weight problems. I always find it amazing that one single, simple eating change has the capacity to make such differences to so many people. So why is food combining so important?

A CHAIN REACTION

Poor food combining is one of the most common mistakes people make with their eating. It's a fundamental error whose consequences are much more wide-ranging and far-reaching than those caused by any single "suspect" food. In fact, poor combining creates problems in which suspect foods then become involved. Other healthy eating methods attempt to put things right by tinkering with what appears to be the "culprit" foods—to little or no effect. The real problem is your food combining.

Poor food combining leads to poor digestion. Poor digestion means toxins are being produced, which interferes at the cellular level with every function of your body and mind at the levels of chemical and bio-electrical activity.

In other words, poor food combining creates and maintains the conditions for problems to develop in your body and mind, or at the very least interferes with your ability to deal with problems from which you may be suffering. It's a deteriorating chain of events that can only worsen as long as you are not combining food well.

- *Excessive toxicity* caused by poor digestion from bad combining means extra demands are being placed on organs that have to neutralize and remove waste materials from your body. Those organs become overworked and more liable to go wrong or become ill. More of your body's energy and resources are needed to keep them working and healthy. Energy and resources you could use better elsewhere.
- *Poor digestion* from poor combining means you'll lack good-quality nutrients for the essential repairs and rebuilding you need. You can't expect to produce a top-quality product if you're using your raw materials badly. The consequences of

poor nutrition is a gradual decline in quality and standards in every area of your body and mind, but particularly in the organs of digestion, some of which become damaged or ill. Even though your body seeks to produce the energy and resources it needs for these problems, it finds them hard to come by in the situation of increasing chaos that is developing within you.

- *Lack of good nutrition* leads to your diet becoming distorted. You want to eat large amounts of some foods because your body is unable to get what it requires from a reasonable amount, but you end up with little benefit and even more toxins because you are unable to digest those foods properly in your deteriorating digestive system. You find yourself eating less and less of other foods because your digestion is unable to deal with them comfortably anymore.

Every day you continue to combine food badly, you remain imprisoned in a situation where the foods you choose add to your problems. Your health will continue to suffer, and your weight will continue to stay beyond your control. In short, your food is your *enemy* instead of your *friend*.

Problems such as those listed above don't just happen; they take time to unfold. Sometimes a great deal of time. Difficulties start to develop only when suitable conditions for dysfunction and disorder arise somewhere in your body or mind. They can progress to become a problem that affects you only by passing through various stages and processes.

At the most basic, cellular level your body and mind work by chemical and bio-electrical processes. By these processes you can function, renew, and repair every part of yourself. If those processes are working well, you will have no problems. If they are interfered with, you will eventually develop a problem. Your food acts on your body and mind in the cells where these chemical and bio-electrical processes are taking place. Your food therefore affects the very levels from which disorder—or good health—arises. It also impacts all the stages through which any health or weight condition must progress to become a difficulty for you.

As soon as you start combining your food well, you stop producing extra toxins. Without excess toxins your body has the chance to clear up toxins that you have already produced. You allow your body to work properly, and to repair and renew itself without interference. You stop creating the conditions which can cause certain foods to become problems.

No wonder, then, so many diverse problems are helped or completely sorted out by correct food combining.

Poor combining, though, is not the only basic eating mistake that has far-reaching consequences for our health, shape, and well-being. Your diet is almost certainly going wrong in other ways as fundamental as food combining and with equally harmful results. Adjusting your eating to address these more comprehensive eating errors rather than targeting specific problem foods offers you the most tremendous potential for improvement with relatively little effort.

One of the great strengths of this diet is that it targets the most destructive and far-reaching of your eating mistakes in ways which give the greatest benefits for the least trouble. That, of course, is why food combining plays such a significant role. As you'll see, however, there are other food strategies and methods which, when added to food combining the *Love Food . . . Lose Weight* way, make it an even more formidable tool with which to turn your food from damaging foe into best friend.

THE KEY TO UNDERSTANDING THE WAY YOU EAT

When your food is a problem for you and you want to know how to turn it into a solution, the most important question you need to ask yourself is: *"Why do I choose to eat what I do?"*

After all, we make choices about what to eat several times a day. So why do so many of us make choices which ultimately harm us? You cannot expect to be able to make better choices and stick to them without finding the answer to this question. No diet is likely to work for you in the long term if it doesn't take into account why you choose the foods you do or why you may be reluctant to change what you choose to eat. You need to know how you can change, so you'll automatically make better choices.

Common sense tells us we're driven to choose the foods we eat by something more than sheer chance, simple convenience, or the pull of our taste buds. Everybody has favorite foods and foods they avoid.

We've all experienced wanting different foods at different times and in different circumstances. Sometimes we prefer salty food, sometimes sweet, on one occasion starchy food, on another a clean, crisp salad. It's not reasonable to believe these choices are completely haphazard. No living thing consumes just anything that's lying around nearby. There's always a purpose that compels them to seek out what they need, a purpose in what they choose to eat and what they reject. There is a purpose in *why* we choose to eat what we do as well.

On this planet of ours, all living things have a certain similarity. Every form of life survives because it is able to successfully organize its inner components, its mental and physical functions, its actions and responses and every other resource it has, to work together. Nothing is redundant; everything is needed and used together to produce and sustain an outer form, inner workings, and behavior that enables each living thing to live, cope, and adapt in the environment it inhabits.

In all living things, including us, every diverse function and process is an essential element which is integrated into a complex working whole. Everything is interconnected—everything functions together—in a continuous process of growth, repair, adaptation, and development. Every component interacts within the whole . . . and the *whole* interacts with the *world*. Self-organization and continuous interaction form the process that enables life to exist: it is the ecological process which starts at conception and ends only at death.

A vital difference separates us from other living things, however. The components integrated into our personal ecologies—the elements which enable us to cope and function as living beings—include those special *mental* and *psychological* qualities that make us human. Not only human—but distinct and individual humans, *unique* human beings.

The process of self-organization which enables you to exist provides you with a uniquely personal ecology. Everything that you are now, and everything that you do now, is the direct result of this ecology. You—as you exist at this moment in time—are a result of your own unique body/mind process, a never-ending process which is going on within you at this very moment.

All living things have another similarity which we share: they take from around them the nutrients they need to enable their particular ecology to work. They digest what food they need to sustain their physical form, and to maintain the complex processes which enable that form to function. So do we.

But because ours is a body/mind ecology, we eat to keep our minds as well as our bodies alive and working. When we choose to eat foods that are bad for us, it therefore has to have something to do with our attempts to make sure our mental and psychological processes can continue to work as we need them to.

There are many clues that confirm this. Look again at the list of problems which are helped by food combining—it's a list of body and mind problems. The various characters I mentioned, whose diets need to differ, are distinguished by personality or temperament as well as physique and activity.

From our own experience and from the information we get from all around us, we know the food we eat is intricately linked with our minds. Foods can cause us to change our minds. Our mood and behavior shift in response to what we eat and drink. Our frame of mind leads us to choose the food that fits our moods.

The old saying "You are what you eat" implies that your food builds you, the entire person, mind and body, personality and form. If you turn that saying around to "You eat what you are," it indicates you choose foods to maintain that entire person. There's something about the person you are which influences you to choose the foods you do.

Yet still we choose foods that harm us—so what is it about how we are as people which can cause us to eat badly?

Perhaps the really unique feature which separates us from other living things is the way our minds contain an internal self-image. Each of us has, from our earliest years, acquired a distinctive way of perceiving ourselves. Our self-image is a construction, built on what we've come to accept about who we are and how we can be in the world, and what we have to do to cope with it. Our self-image is closely related to all our experiences and acts as a frame of reference. We use our self-image to assess what's happening to us, what we should do in any situation, how we should act, what we believe we can achieve, and so on. We often use it without knowing we are doing so and without realizing the implications, because our self-image is held in the form of attitudes, beliefs, assumptions, memories, and conclusions in our unconscious minds. It gives us a way of seeing everything in the world around us in a context which we can understand and use to help us get by. It has a tremendous influence over us and has immense implications for our health, shape, and happiness.

Your inner self-image is the basis for the way you feel about yourself and what you think you are capable of. It therefore influences the choices you make in every area of your life—but its role goes far beyond your mind. Our very nature as living beings means our self-image is inextricably linked, not only with the other parts of our mind such as thoughts, feelings, and decisions, but with our body and our behavior as well.

The framework of your self-image leads you to see yourself and the world in the unique way you do, and to think and feel about it as you do. Your thoughts and feelings affect *every* part of your body. Emotions are a full-body experience; you feel them in your body as well as in your head. Anger "makes your blood boil," fear "makes your bowels turn to water," love "makes your heart beat faster," happiness "makes you feel as light as air" . . . and so on.

Your self-image is involved in every action your body takes and every function that occurs within it. It is, in fact, around your self-image that the entire workings of your body and mind are organized. Your self-image orchestrates and conducts *what* you are and *how* you are.

Our self-image is at the core of the processes which enable us to be the person we believe we are and how we need to be. Our self-image acts to keep us alive in the image we have of ourselves—we human beings aren't just organized to stay alive. We're organized by our inner self-image to stay alive *as the person we believe we should be.* Ultimately, our body and mind and all that they do are subordinate to our self-image.

Everything about us, then, is organized to sustain the deepest inner beliefs we have about the way we are.

So what causes us to do something no other living thing does—consistently eat foods which harm us?

The answer lies in your self-image—as you would expect. Your self-image governs how you eat in two distinctive ways. First, because it orchestrates the body and mind, your self-image is the ultimate influence on your choice of foods to maintain that body/mind. You are what you eat . . . and you *eat* what you *are* . . . and what you are is *what your self-image makes you.*

Second, we are creatures of preference—we prefer to feel in control of our lives. We prefer to see ourselves and feel and think about ourselves in ways that do not cause us to be confused. We prefer to retain the self-image we best understand and suppress any aspects of it which confuse us.

If your self-image were perfect—if there were such a thing as a perfect self-image—you would be perfectly healthy, perfectly shaped, and you would instinctively eat perfectly.

But what happens if parts of your inner self-image aren't compatible with others? What if you feel yourself to be one way, but have accepted—because others have told you so—that you are something different? What if your reasoning tells you things ought to be *one* way, but at the insistence of others you've accepted them as *another*? What if early on in life, helpless and vulnerable, you acquired beliefs about yourself from different but equally influential sources, beliefs that contradicted one another or were in conflict with your instinctive needs and desires? What kind of self-image will you have developed from such beginnings?

You may be aware of parts of your self-image which you do not like to think about. Perhaps you already know things about yourself which are not how you would like them to be. You may be aware of thoughts, feelings, behavior, and reactions to events you would prefer not to have.

It's characteristics such as these, arising not from flaws or mistakes, but from inconsistencies and incongruities in your self-image, that ultimately create bad eating choices . . . and all that results from them.

Many foods have a direct effect on our minds. The chemistry they create in our brains enables us to think in a particular way. Our diet, then, naturally tends toward those foods which help us see, feel, and think about ourselves in the ways we most readily accept is true (or find most useful). We tend *not* to eat what makes us see ourselves and our lives in ways we don't accept (or don't find useful).

You Choose to Eat What Helps You to Be the Person You Need to Be

You eat in ways that support most what you have come to accept as yourself, and how you need to be. But you do so at the cost of what you could be and at the cost of your long-term health.

Particular foods give us access to one kind of thinking or feeling over another—that is to say, access to one way of seeing ourselves and the world over another. In sports, for example, it's no surprise athletes use their diet not just as a means of providing energy and improving muscle and joint quality, but also as a way of maintaining their best mental attitude.

For the rest of us, the most obvious foods which affect personality and mood are coffee, tea, chocolate, and alcohol. But fatty foods, protein-rich foods, or starchy foods have also been identified as being able to affect depression, anger, mood, memory, alertness, and sensitivity to pain. Foods can enhance a feeling of well-being and suppress anger and anxiety. They can boost self-confidence and reduce irritability and unhappiness.

Comfort eating is a habit that's particularly common among women. Eating a lot of sweet and starchy foods enables the brain to raise its level of the chemical serotonin, a naturally occurring antidepressant. Raising serotonin levels produces feelings of greater confidence and optimism and reduces moodiness, sadness, irritability, and sensitivity to pain. Low serotonin can predispose you to suffer more sadness, pessimism, anxieties about inadequacies you believe you have, or doubts about certain life situations you are in.

If you're a comfort eater, in order to sustain your preferred self-image and the thoughts and feelings that go with it, you are inclined to eat comfort foods more and more frequently until their use becomes habitual.

We all know a high intake of sweet and starchy foods, especially when other foods are excluded, leads to weight gain and eventually obesity. These foods also disrupt the environment of your digestive tract, causing bloating in the intestines, distension of the abdomen, fluid retention, and setting up the conditions suitable for yeast infections. In addition, your digestion becomes less efficient, requiring you to eat more comfort food in order to produce the "right" kind of feelings. Your body processes become less and less able to service the needs of all the other organs, glands, and vital systems from a deteriorating diet and inefficient digestion. Your body/mind struggles more and more to maintain an equilibrium.

This increasing chaos establishes the background for one health problem after another. It's the insidious process, occurring over many months or even years, which involves bad eating but which arises from a poor inner self-image. What you notice are increasing weight, mood, and behavior changes and a slowly deteriorating general health.

If you thought you chose what you eat simply because of your taste buds or because of a hunger response, you must see now that you should think again. All your choices are driven, in one way or another, by the influence of your self-image, and *no* self-image is perfect.

Your diet ultimately cannot succeed unless you change those parts of your self-image that will hinder you, and continue to influence you to eat in ways that harm you. You must be able to alter how you see yourself so the ways you think and feel about yourself become influences to choose foods that are good for you.

Changing your self-image is a skill that can be learned. One of the most important aspects of *Love Food . . . Lose Weight* is that it teaches you to alter your self-image, using simple but powerful methods.

Your self-image is a construction. Most of it was given to you piece by piece by other people who were influential in your life. You built other parts of your inner self on your own, from your conclusions and assumptions in response to what others communicated to you. You can rebuild your self-image at any time you want, to be whatever you choose. The consequences for your body/mind will be as far-reaching as any diet, but together with *Love Food . . . Lose Weight* the effects are wonderful.

And that brings us to the most interesting question of all so far—a question only you can answer. If changing your self-image would make so much difference to your health, your weight, and your life as a whole—*"How do you want to see yourself?"*

How Not to Diet

Most diets don't produce the goods.

It's true that even on an unsuitable diet you may start out by losing a bit of weight. You might find yourself slimmer and even a little healthier. But inevitably you end up back where you started. Worse still, you often end up a few steps behind where you began. A bad diet can ultimately diminish your self-esteem, cause you to feel and look worse than before, and send you sliding into even worse eating habits than you had. When a bad diet lets you down, trying again becomes more difficult.

Most diets fail because they are too extreme and attempt too much too quickly.

Over many years your body and mind, orchestrated by your self-image, have worked together to establish a delicate equilibrium. As best they can, they have created a fairly serviceable process for coping with your life experiences and for keeping your body working.

But it's a precarious harmony. The bad eating, excess weight, poor shape, or deteriorating health testifies to how fragile the organization of all your inner and outer resources really is, and how much it needs improving.

What do you think is likely to happen if that shaky stability is suddenly disturbed by a radical change in an established eating pattern that, despite its unsuitability, underpins the entire complex system?

Chaos!

One, two, perhaps a few weeks at the most, of enthusiastic activity to keep the diet going is followed by a plunge into demotivation, self-anger, guilt, cravings, and failure, as your entire body/mind process is thrown into disarray. And that disarray brings about more problems when a frail self-esteem is damaged further and adds to the contradictions of an already poor self-image.

Vary an established eating pattern too drastically or too rapidly, and it can be more than counterproductive: it can be harmful. The effects are not always immediate; they can continue to echo for a long time afterward. Like knocking down the first domino in a row . . .

Another way of dieting that fails more often than not is the kind that fiddles around with the minutiae of your food intake.

Apart from there not being sufficient valid reasons to think that removing or including any one food or type of food is going to produce the effect you expect, you can't be sure if the food you are concerned about *is* the one that needs attention.

Suddenly removing a food that's regularly featured in your diet, or suddenly *including* large amounts of one that hasn't, has similar effects of any other drastic alteration to your eating pattern. These are distress, ultimate failure, and potential harm because of the after-effects in your complex body/mind/self-image interaction.

Not convinced? Try eating a very high-fiber diet when you're not used to much in your diet and see how you fare. Try a sudden shift to raw foods or try giving up sugar, caffeine, or bread if you've been using them every day. Notice not just what happens in your body but what happens to your thoughts and feelings!

Altering the intake of a specific food in your diet invariably has a marginal effect on what you want to improve, especially when there are other problems with your eating that are much more serious and far-reaching. Minor adjustments to salt or sugar intake, for instance, are difficult to do, and a lot of effort for little or no return *if you are still combining badly*. Of course, if you have good reason to believe you are at risk from a food, you must reduce your intake, but otherwise you should put your efforts where they will do more good.

How many people do you know (and maybe you count yourself among them) who while on a diet have described irritability, moodiness, irrational feelings, melancholy, lack of energy, disorientation, and an intense desire to give up? Is it any wonder?

Your self-image reacts to any disturbance in your body/mind by causing you to retrench into old habits of behavior. The more dramatic the disturbance, the more emphatic the self-protection and reinforcing of past patterns.

The best diet gets the foundations right first.

Poor use of foods, overeating, poor health, poor weight control, are all symptoms stemming from the main problem, namely disorganization in the body/mind process. As that is restored by the use of food combining and the other strategies that make up *Love Food . . . Lose Weight*, you'll find that many of those symptoms disappear. If, after using this diet for a while, you're still being bothered by a problem or if you want to speed your changes up a bit, you can use one of the many special techniques you'll find later on in the book.

THE ESSENTIAL ELEMENTS
OF SUCCESSFUL DIETING

If your diet is going to be successful, it *must* work in harmony with your body and mind.

If your diet conflicts with the ways your mind and body act together to help you stay alive and cope in the world, then you are bound to cause more problems than you have now. The cells of your body are constantly dying off and being replaced. With the exception of your brain, you are completely rebuilt approximately every two years. Rebuilt but not necessarily *renewed*, because the "new you" can actually be a poorer replica of the old. At each cycle exists the possibility, if the materials and conditions for your renewal deteriorate, of flaws or weaknesses being created. This can generate fresh health and weight problems, or make old problems worse.

The renewal of our body is affected by several factors that are within your control. For one, the quality of the environment where cellular renewal takes place. For another, the quality of the essential materials from which your new cells are made or with which you create the environment in which your cells have to function.

Did you know that your body prioritizes how it uses its energy and resources? If it faces a crisis, say an injury or illness, it neglects other, less essential work elsewhere in order to address the problem that poses the greatest threat. Constant crises lead to *persistent neglect* and, inevitably, *more* crises.

The foremost agent at your disposal for influencing these factors is your diet. A successful diet is one that encourages and supports the natural process of cellular regeneration. A poor diet taxes the digestive system and creates excessive amounts of toxins. That toxicity affects your body's environment at the level of renewal, resulting in poor quality of essential materials for renewal and function. A poor diet results in damage to and reduction of the efficiency of the organs of digestion that must produce new cellular material, and it does the same to the organs that cleanse your body of toxic material. It produces crises that have to be dealt with at the cost of neglect elsewhere. *A bad diet drives your body into a downward spiral of deterioration.*

A good diet does not overstress your digestive system; it encourages it to work more effectively. A good diet does not produce more toxins than you can deal with comfortably; it enables you to progressively get rid of toxins that have already accumulated in your body. A good diet improves the environment where cellular activity regenerates your body; step by step you become better and better. I have an expression for the beneficial influence a good diet exerts: I call it a *positive disturbance*. All disturbances create a reaction. A positive disturbance provokes your body's natural impulse to adapt in a productive way. A good diet prompts adaptations away from illness, poor weight control, and bad self-image, towards health, trimness, and a good feeling about who you are.

One key to a successful diet is to take care about how you use your *mind* as well as your *mouth*. A successful diet creates the conditions for a change of mind as well as a change of body. This means it will act moderately—not violently—and enable you to create more self-esteem, and help you get used to the new thoughts and feelings that go with them, at the same time as you get used to your new body. A good diet is one that makes a new reality more accessible, not one that causes you to retrench into old habits.

Your mind takes time to change. If it's given the opportunity to accept the idea of a new you gradually, as you proceed, it will help you subconsciously, continually, and potently. The right *diet*, used skillfully, enables you to alter your self-image into a powerful force for health and personal improvement. The right *self-image*, built skillfully, enables you to alter your diet into a powerful force for health and personal improvement.

I advise my clients *not* to change their diet without also addressing what is one of the driving forces behind their poor eating in the first place: their *self-image*.

And you thought your diet was just a matter of how much you ate!

The most successful diet works with, not against, the natural dynamics of your body/mind process. It restores harmony and proper function in progressive steps. And as you progress, you'll discover a fascinating phenomenon: the "moment of recovery."

Most of the problems from which you suffer are the result of a lengthy process during which your body and mind were diverted from the best they might have achieved by inconsistencies in your inner self-image. When problems arise in these circumstances, they do so because some aspect of your body or mind, in the ever-changing process of what you are, reaches a point of breakdown or distress, and something has to give way. Often what occurs is a payoff that enables you and your body to continue to function—but in a weaker or compromised state. These are moments of loss and decline to which your poor eating has contributed.

With a good diet you will create a situation that produces a complete contrast to these unhappy occasions. Moments when you realize you have evolved into a better state of health, or achieved a fresh and more enabling way of seeing yourself, or when you suddenly feel a freeing-up of some part of your body or a release from a limiting thought or emotion.

These "moments of recovery" are unpredictable, occurring when you reach a natural milestone of improvement in one or other of the diverse elements of your body and mind. At such instances you cross a physical, biochemical, or psychological threshold and achieve spontaneous shifts that are healing, joyful, and enabling in a multitude of ways. Be aware and savor them—they're fun, they're wonderful, and they can be truly moving.

FOOD COMBINING THE
LOVE FOOD . . . LOSE WEIGHT WAY

Of all the methods of dieting you could choose, food combining fulfills virtually all the essentials of the perfect diet. Our method of food combining makes these essentials even more accessible and effective.

To be effectively digested, each food you eat needs the right chemical environment in your body. Combining foods badly means one of the foods, at least, will mix with the wrong chemicals. The result is a poorly digested meal and more toxins than necessary as by-products.

Poorly digested foods, as you now realize, are the first steps in a string of consequences that lead to a lot of problems.

There are two types of food that need quite different environments for complete and effective digestion. They are foods rich in protein and foods rich in starch or sugar (the carbohydrates).

Put them together in any meal and neither is digested properly, so it makes sense to keep them apart. The one single rule of food combining in this diet is:

Don't eat proteins and carbohydrates so they are present in your stomach at the same time.

Every other food combining recommendation is subject to some exceptions, conditions, or reinterpretation—except this one. It is nonnegotiable!

The only two things you have to know now are: first, how to change your habit of putting proteins and carbohydrates together in your meals; and second, how to find out which foods are proteins and which are carbohydrates. Don't worry about this, I'm going to make it easy for you. You've taken a while to get here, just take a little longer to get used to the idea of better combining, and then I'll show you how easy it can be.

Now, those of you with a bent for self-defeat will already be looking for the get-out clauses and mistaken interpretations that will enable you to mess this up.

Seriously, there are people like that. That's why so many diets get so complicated. By trying to cross all the t's and dot all the i's, and close all the loopholes, their instructions start to look like a knitting pattern for a hot-air balloon or a manual for a mainframe computer.

You're going to have to make up your mind—and now is as good a time as any—that:

- You are going to make this diet work if humanly possible (I've made it work and I'm human, so that takes care of that!) *and*
- You are going to interpret the instructions in the *best* way you can to make the diet work—you are *not* going to use them as an excuse to fail.

Please take a moment to think about that before you continue.

So: proteins and carbohydrates . . . not in your stomach together . . . don't eat them in the same meal or too close together . . . Remember? And what *is* too close together? (You can see how complicated it could get, can't you? Each answer can mean another question!) The answers to questions like this—if they aren't clear from my instructions—are to be found in two places:

First, in your own head. What do *you* think too close together means? If you want to mess up your diet, you'll say five minutes. Otherwise it will vary from a couple of hours to something like eight depending on how much you know about your body and how keen you are to stick to the diet. Eight is exaggerated caution and rather on the self-punishing side. Two is perhaps a little optimistic, but not too far off—even if you sometimes eat conflicting foods within two hours of each other, it would be better than eating them together. Try for about four hours and you're OK. Most people do get hungry about every four hours.

Sometimes an accurate answer to a question about diet isn't possible, and isn't what you really *need* anyway. Sometimes what you really need is the confidence that comes from believing you're doing the right thing. With some diets you get a whole heap of data dumped on you when all you really want is to know if you're doing OK.

So you're doing OK if you allow two hours between incompatible foods, but four hours is best. One person at least, reading this, has just thought, "I'll do three." That's good. It's better than five minutes or even two hours.

The other place to find an answer to questions is in a medical textbook. It'll probably yield a general answer for the average time it takes the optimum system to digest each type of food.

Do you have the optimum digestive system? I know I don't, for one. There's no such thing! Stomach acid, enzyme secretion, gallbladder function, all vary from one person to another. Stick with me and I'll show you how to make decisions that will work for you; I'll show you a better way than trying to eat by a rule book.

How about identifying what foods are which types? Simple. There is a directory at the back of this book. Just look up the food in the alphabetical list, and it will tell you all you need to know. You'll soon find, though, that you'll be able to make a fair stab at recognizing foods by their character and where they come from. After a few days you won't need to look them up at all. The little charts that follow will help you, too.

Remember, though, *your intention is the best foundation for your success*. Success will not come from trying to follow rigid rules or from the clutter of too much information at the wrong time. It will come from your intention to make your diet work. All your good efforts will not be destroyed either if you guess and are wrong occasionally, as long as you check out your guess and make sure you don't keep repeating the same mistake over and over again because you couldn't be bothered.

Eat thoughtfully, and you'll surprise yourself with what you know.

PROTEINS—A MEMORY AID
"Proteins Are Nuts That Eat Seeds"

(Proteins are mainly animal products, plus nuts, seeds, and soya.)

Animal Products	Non-Animal Products
Fish • Game • Meats • Beef Innards • Poultry • Shellfish • Cheeses • Eggs	Coconut • Nuts • Seeds • Soy • Soy products

SPECIAL CASES
Milk: use milk in small amounts only
Yogurt: easy to digest and can be combined with any other food including fruits

So that's proteins in a nutshell. Proteins are marked P in the directory at the back. Proteins can be combined with other proteins in a meal but not with carbohydrates.

CARBOHYDRATES—A MEMORY AID
"Carbohydrates Can Be Starchy or Sweet But Are Never Stuffy"

(Carbohydrates are mainly foods that are starchy or sweet. If you can mash it like potatoes or make it into a flour, it's a carbohydrate. You mustn't use them as stuffing for proteins, though, because proteins and carbohydrates shouldn't be mixed.)

Gluten Cereals	Beans/Peas
Barley • Oats • Rye • Wheat	Beans/Peas (dried) • Chickpeas • Lentils (all) • Peanuts
Non-Gluten Grains	**Vegetables**
Buckwheat • Millet • Rice	Corn • Potatoes

SPECIAL CASES
Flours made from any of the above

Sugars
All sugars, honey, molasses, maple syrup, etc.

Lentils and beans are good sources of proteins for vegetarians, but they're mainly starchy in character and are generally difficult to digest except in small quantities. Carbohydrates can be combined with other carbohydrates in a meal but not with proteins. Carbohydrates are marked C in the directory at the back.

Now all you need to know is what to do with the foods that are left. Most of them can be mixed with either proteins or carbohydrates, so I call them Mix With Any Foods.

MIX WITH ANY FOODS

Vegetables, Salads, and Vegetable Juices
All low and non-starchy vegetables and salads unless listed elsewhere. If in doubt, check the directory at the back for a complete list. Vegetables, salads, and vegetable juices combine well with either proteins or carbohydrates.

Oils and Fats	Condiments and Flavorings
Butter • Cream • Drippings Fish oils • Nut oils • Olive oil • Suet Vegetable oils Oils and fats should be used sparingly and special care taken when combining with carbohydrates if slimming is a concern. Oils and fats mix with *either* proteins *or* carbohydrates.	Condiments • Herbs • Spices Natural flavorings Including: chilies, garlic, pepper, salt, vinegars, pickles, soy sauce, mustard, natural essences—see directory for a more complete list. All condiments and flavorings can be combined with any other food if used sparingly. Fresh herbs can be used more generously.

You'll see all the Mix With Any Foods marked M/A in the directory at the back. I expect you're already beginning to see what sort of meals you could make by following these guidelines. If that means you're also concerned about things like when you can eat french fries if you can't have them with steak, stay with me and I'll show you that there are other ways to enjoy fries.

Some of you reading this may be getting ready to cut and run right now, but believe me, this will all come as naturally as falling off a log after a few days. Do you remember learning something new, say driving a car, or knitting, or working a computer? The feelings of confusion when you're starting to learn a new skill or enterprise are the same whatever the subject—head in a whirl with all that new stuff to remember, body feeling all awkward, hands like bunches of bananas. But it all feels so normal after a short while, doesn't it, that you wonder what all the fuss was about? Get in the car, check the gear stick, and start up without thinking; knit one pearl one as you chat away; tap your fingers waiting for the microchips to "please get on with it."

Just give yourself time to get used to the idea of food combining—and some leeway to make a few mistakes.

So all that's left now are the fruits.

FRUIT

Fresh Fruits, Dried Fruits, and Fruit Juices
Apples Apricots Bananas Berries (all) Blackcurrants Cherries Currants Elderberry Grapes Guava Kiwi Lychees Mango Papaya Passion fruit Peaches Pears Persimmon Pineapple Prunes Redcurrants All dried fruits

Fruits, generally speaking, don't mix well with anything else. They nip through your stomach and into other parts of your digestive system so quickly. If they get held up—especially with proteins—they can cause problems. There *are* ways of mixing fruits with other foods. There are even ways that seem to go contrary to old Dr. Hay's rules, but not for you right now. For now the advice is:

Eat fruits mixed only with fruits, and don't mix melon with anything but other melon.

The way you'll be food combining in a few months from now will be different. When you first start, however, you are learning new ideas and trying to break old habits. The best way to do that is to methodically follow a plan and stick closely to the food-combining rules so you won't become confused. You can leave the exceptions and subtleties until later.

It's at the start of food combining that you'll learn most, get the best and fastest responses, and acquire the best habits. Don't deprive yourself of that brief, important time by looking for variations just yet.

Later on, I'll show you how to bend all the rules, make reasonable reinterpretations to suit special circumstances, and even why it's OK to break the rules of food combining completely once in a while. But modifications like that work best after you've become used to basic combining.

That's all you need to know about combining your food for now.

Oh, yes! I need to say something about drinks.

What to drink with meals, in the context of food combining, is not so much a matter of what combines well as what effect the fluid will have on your digestion. Particularly on the digestion of proteins, which require a strong acid environment in your stomach. Anyway, it's quite straightforward.

Wine, champagne, black coffee and tea, and vegetable juices are all right with any food. Spirits in modest amounts shouldn't be too much of a problem, either, but are best avoided if weight loss is desired. It's best not to drink water or fruit juices with any meal, and any gassy drinks like beer should be avoided, too.

OK, that is definitely it.

The following is a quick reference chart to show you at a glance which foods mix and which do not.

By the way, do you remember what foods are proteins and which are carbohydrates?

PROTEINS ARE NUTS THAT EAT SEEDS!
(Animal products, soy, nuts, and seeds)
CARBOHYDRATES CAN BE STARCHY OR SWEET BUT ARE NEVER STUFFY!
(Cereals, potatoes, rice, beans and lentils, peanuts)
[Just checking!]

YOUR QUICK REFERENCE GUIDE
TO EASY FOOD COMBINING

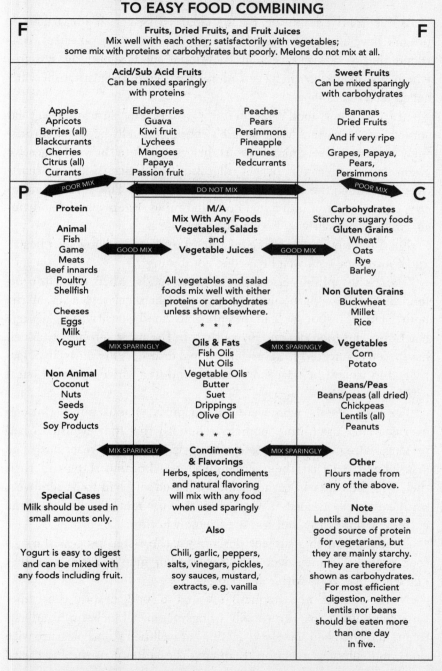

F   **Fruits, Dried Fruits, and Fruit Juices**   **F**
Mix well with each other; satisfactorily with vegetables;
some mix with proteins or carbohydrates but poorly. Melons do not mix at all.

Acid/Sub Acid Fruits
Can be mixed sparingly
with proteins

Apples	Elderberries	Peaches
Apricots	Guava	Pears
Berries (all)	Kiwi fruit	Persimmons
Blackcurrants	Lychees	Pineapple
Cherries	Mangoes	Prunes
Citrus (all)	Papaya	Redcurrants
Currants	Passion fruit	

Sweet Fruits
Can be mixed sparingly
with carbohydrates

Bananas
Dried Fruits

And if very ripe

Grapes, Papaya,
Pears,
Persimmons

P   ◀ POOR MIX   ◀ DO NOT MIX ▶   ◀ POOR MIX ▶   **C**

Protein

M/A
Mix With Any Foods
Vegetables, Salads
and
Vegetable Juices

Carbohydrates
Starchy or sugary foods
Gluten Grains
Wheat
Oats
Rye
Barley

Animal
Fish
Game   ◀ GOOD MIX
Meats
Beef innards
Poultry
Shellfish

GOOD MIX ▶

All vegetables and salad
foods mix well with either
proteins or carbohydrates
unless shown elsewhere.

* * *

Non Gluten Grains
Buckwheat
Millet
Rice

Cheeses
Eggs
Milk
Yogurt   ◀ MIX SPARINGLY

Oils & Fats
Fish Oils
Nut Oils
Vegetable Oils
Butter
Suet
Drippings
Olive Oil

MIX SPARINGLY ▶

Vegetables
Corn
Potato

Non Animal
Coconut
Nuts
Seeds
Soy
Soy Products

* * *

Beans/Peas
Beans/peas (all dried)
Chickpeas
Lentils (all)
Peanuts

◀ MIX SPARINGLY

Condiments
& Flavorings
Herbs, spices, condiments
and natural flavoring
will mix with any food
when used sparingly

MIX SPARINGLY ▶

Other
Flours made from
any of the above.

Special Cases
Milk should be used in
small amounts only.

Yogurt is easy to digest
and can be mixed with
any foods including fruit.

Also

Chili, garlic, peppers,
salts, vinegars, pickles,
soy sauces, mustard,
extracts, e.g. vanilla

Note
Lentils and beans are a
good source of protein
for vegetarians, but
they are mainly starchy.
They are therefore
shown as carbohydrates.
For most efficient
digestion, neither
lentils nor beans
should be eaten more
than one day
in five.

ONE IN FIVE—YOUR SECRET STRATEGY

While food combining comes close to being an ideal diet, it doesn't have all the answers. Here is a very simple yet powerful technique that you won't find in traditional food-combining systems, which will give your diet even more of an edge over any other. It's called *food rotation*.

At its simplest, food rotation is a way of making sure you don't eat some foods too often. Most people's eating gradually becomes surprisingly habitual. A very monotonous diet can deplete the vital digestive chemistry needed for proper digestion of foods that are being overused, much the same as bad combining does. This results in toxicity, compromise of individual body and mind systems, and disorganization of the underlying body/mind processes.

Food rotation is, therefore, as important to improving your health and controlling your weight as food combining.

There's something else as well: some foods, when eaten too often, can provoke particularly unpleasant chemical responses in the body. These responses can manifest as food sensitivities, allergic reactions, and food dependencies that, in the most serious instances, have been connected to severe emotional disorders in adults, hyperactivity and violent behavior in children, and to a whole raft of physical problems.

I've had clients who were caught in a vicious circle through overuse. They used some foods so frequently that they eventually had to stop eating them completely because of adverse reactions. The result has been that their remaining foods became staples in their diet, and then they in turn became overused and had to be removed, until eventually their diet was limited to very few foods and became extremely unhealthy, not to say extremely boring.

Literature on this subject describes a three-step process. First, a food provokes some adverse physical and/or mental reaction, rather like cow's milk does with most babies.

Next, repeated and frequent use of the food, despite the earlier unpleasant reactions, eventually brings about a biochemical adjustment, and the bad food elicits feelings of well-being and pleasure with no serious physical reaction. Reducing the amount of the food used causes physical and emotional withdrawal symptoms. Frequency and amount of the food is therefore increased—dependency is established. This step can last months or years.

Finally, increased frequency no longer induces a pleasurable response. Full-blown allergic reactions and severe physical or mental disturbance are experienced when the food is used. The sufferer rejects the food and seeks another substance that will make them feel better.

The phenomenon is called *masked* food allergic response.

Without your being aware of it, food overuse may already have distorted the balance of your entire diet. This can happen with more than one food at a time. It can arise at any stage, for any of the foods involved. It can be extremely severe or simply a minor irritation in your life. To the sufferer who doesn't make the link with their food, these problems may seem to have no discernible cause. At whatever stage, however apparently innocuous the effect, food overuse is both indicator and cause of health problems affecting your entire body/mind system. The good news is—it can be easily managed.

Foods most likely to be or become a problem are those you eat a lot of or use daily, especially if it's a food used *more* than once a day.

If you don't think you have habit foods or potentially dependent foods, just consider, right now, giving up coffee, tea, cola, bread, biscuits, chocolate, sugar, salt, cheese or milk, or any other food that you might be using daily. The very thought of doing so may be traumatic!

Common symptoms of masked food allergic response include:

- Unusual weight fluctuation
- Bloating after meals
- Headaches
- Sweating, not from exercise
- Puffiness (fluid retention)
- Abdominal discomfort
- Bowel problems
- Nasal discharge or sinus problems
- Palpitations after food

Food rotation can help all these conditions. It means:

> **Foods which may become a problem from overuse should be eaten one day only in any five days.**

In the directory these foods are marked * and referred to as "1 in 5" foods.

The most obvious question is, Which foods are they? So you don't have to keep looking at the directory, remember as a general rule 1 in 5 foods are the proteins, the carbohydrates, and some foods you eat daily or almost daily, but don't include fresh fruits or any Mix With Any vegetables or salads.

I can almost hear your gasps! So let me quickly reassure you this *isn't* nearly as difficult as it might seem.

For a start, not many people eat the same protein daily, and meat protein sensitivity is very rare (do you eat chicken or pork every day? Almost certainly not). Also, the rule applies to individual foods, not entire groups, so although you may be overusing a single kind of nut, for example, you can easily *change* to eating a different type of nut every day and *still* comply with the 1 in 5 rule. The same applies to different types of fish—you can have fish every day, as long as it is of different kinds. You can have different kinds of meat or poultry, and if you choose to have cow's-milk cheese one day, sheep's the next, and goat's cheese the next, you're still within the 1 in 5 rule. How's *that* for a rule that invites you to eat anything you want?

While plenty of people do eat several carbohydrates every day, you can probably imagine the benefits you'll get for your health and weight by controlling your intake of potatoes, bread and pasta (both wheat), and rice. Food rotation is the way to do it—*without* giving up any of them. Just make them 1 in 5 foods.

When you analyze food rotation carefully, there are actually only a few foods which most people need to consider as potential problems. The most common are the cereals and particularly wheat products (especially bread), soy products, eggs, cow's-milk dairy products (especially cheese), yeast extracts, potatoes, chocolate, and caffeine products (coffee, tea, cola, etc.). These foods can have potent effects.

They can alter what's happening in your body or mind in dramatic ways.

Think about how caffeine, alcohol, fatty foods, carbohydrates, salt, and sugar can affect you. Consider what they do to brain function, mood, bowel movement, fluid balance in your body, pancreatic activity, personality, and energy levels. These foods affect you powerfully, and by using them too often you can be creating what I term a "function debt." In that situation the workings of your body or mind are modified because foods are constantly imposing themselves.

Let me explain. Nature is very economical. It won't waste energy and resources where it doesn't have to. If you regularly use foods which simulate or stimulate your body's normal processes, your body systems will eventually come to accept the effect and adapt to it. Your body can consequently become *dependent* on a food and reduce its own ability to produce the same effect, or it can be provoked into overactivity by a food. Either way the normal healthy working of the systems which make up your body and mind becomes distorted.

Think about it like this. If you hurt your leg and needed a crutch to get around on, the muscles in the damaged leg would shrink and weaken from lack of use. When your leg is healed, if you don't let go of the crutch and start using the leg, it will *remain weak*. What do you think would happen if you were unprepared or afraid to give up the crutch even after your leg was able to be used again?

Yes, you'd lose more and more and more tone in the muscles and mobility in your leg. As time passed, more and more effort would be required to restore normal strength and function. Your leg would effectively have given up its place as a genuine part of your functioning body—to the crutch. This is nature's way of adapting to circumstances and prioritizing its resources on your behalf. It happens with powerful foods you could be using—like crutches—too often in your diet.

The 1 in 5 rule makes sure you vary your diet and don't eat anything too often. That will automatically mean you are breaking the cycle of any food you may be becoming allergic to or dependent on, and enables your body to restore itself to full health without dietary crutches.

If you do have an allergy or dependency without realizing it, 1 in 5 also means you will get a chance to positively identify any food you're having a problem with at the same time as you are reducing its harmful effects.

The rule is called 1 in 5 because it takes up to five days for your body to eliminate the effects of regular doses of any food to which you may have become sensitive. During the first few days you may identify a food by craving for it. After five days you can identify it if you notice a definite reaction when you eat it again.

The 1 in 5 rule allows your body to readapt and restore functions suppressed by the function debt. It enables you to gradually throw away dietary crutches and bring the wholeness back to your body/mind process.

There are benefits to be had from food rotation other than the obvious ones to your health and weight. For a start you'll have to discover some alternatives to the foods you've come to rely on. That means you have a chance to give your diet some variation, which will make it both *more* interesting and *more* enjoyable, not less.

Another really worthwhile plus from rotation is what I call BFDs. A BFD is a Best Food Day. If you are going to be eating some foods you really like on only one day in five, what you do is make sure you get the best quality, the most enjoyable, and the most special of each of these foods that you can on that one day you are going to eat it—because you're not going to eat it again in the next four days. When you eat a food too often, the tendency is to take it for granted and even eat poor-quality examples of that food. Eaten less frequently, foods can become special and enjoyable again. Familiarity brings contempt— 1 in 5 brings *contentment*.

So on your wheat BFD you have your favorite pasta and, if you want it, your favorite bread. On a cheese BFD, get your favorite cheeses and so on. Suddenly, every day can become a treat day. So don't despair over the "loss" of your favorite foods: food rotation will be something to look forward to. You won't be deprived and needn't be disappointed!

It's easy when reading a book like this, where all the information comes thick and fast, to get a little overwhelmed at the prospect of making it all work. Very soon I'm going to give you all the help and practical advice you'll need so that even if you can't do this with your eyes shut, you'll only have to have them half open to be on the right track.

My advice with food rotation is to rotate the most common habit foods first—wheat foods, potatoes, cheese, soy if you use it a lot, and leave anything else until you've been a combiner and rotator for at least a couple of months.

By then you'll be feeling good, looking good, and ready to consider some of the other methods in this book that will help you to look and feel even better. Then you can think about whether rotating other foods may be useful and something you'd like to try—and again, I'll give you ways of making it easy to rotate even the most addictive foods.

> If you find it difficult to rotate one or other of the main habit foods to the 1 in 5 rule because they cause withdrawal symptoms, reduce them to 1 in 2 or 1 in 3, and slowly withdraw from them until you are eating them only 1 in 5.

Again I want to stress: don't worry about trying to remember all this. You'll get all the help you need later, in the form of menus, to show you how to rotate and combine your food, and recipes that will tempt you into trying foods you may not yet use in your diet. You'll have strategies for easing into combining and rotation so gently and effectively that you'll find yourself doing what you need to with very little effort and a lot of enjoyment!

BEWARE WHEAT!

Wheat is your Number One food enemy.

Does it surprise you that I should be so damning about a food that's so common? You see, that's the problem—it is *so* common in our lives. Wheat exemplifies the problem of food overuse. Nearly everyone eats it without thinking and often without knowing because it turns up in so many prepared foods. Virtually all fast foods include it, and yet the only real health question about wheat in people's minds is "whole wheat or refined?"

"To eat or not to eat wheat?"—that ought to be the question.

Wheat is seriously overused in our society. Think about all the bread, pasta, cakes, biscuits, breakfast cereals, filler in sausages, soups, and sweets you're exposed to every day. Then add the pies, pizzas, flans, pastries, sandwiches, and burgers. Wheat covers fish, chicken, and turkey. It's filled with jam, cheese, and umpteen other unsuitable substances, and if you pause for a moment, I'm sure you can think of even more foods where wheat is involved.

Not surprisingly, most people eat wheat in some form every day and often several times a day, with unfortunate consequences. Yet they have little reason to suspect wheat as being involved in their health or weight problems.

If any one food plays a major part in our society's trend toward overweight, it's probably wheat. I have not come across a single person who, if they've taken my advice to alter their use of wheat, hasn't benefited from a real weight and health improvement as a result.

That's a one hundred percent response to one simple change in diet.

I've seen people become less moody and resolve sinus conditions that have affected them for decades by controlling their wheat intake. People lose four pounds' weight in one week just by not eating wheat for that time. I've personally experienced and seen others gain three to four pounds' weight overnight after eating an occasional meal containing wheat, and lose it again during the following forty-eight hours without wheat. Some people's abdomens bloat like a football after a single wheat meal, and they've solved the problem by limiting wheat in their diet. I've seen people whose control of wheat was an important part of lessening severe Chronic Fatigue Syndrome or simple pains in their joints and muscles. There are even serious scientific suggestions that the constant illness—nausea, vomiting, headaches, fatigue, palpitations, and eczema—which plagued Charles Darwin for nearly forty years, was actually caused by a masked food allergy to wheat.*

---

*"Cooking up a storm." Gamlin, L., *New Scientist*, July 8, 1989.

Wheat is a major culprit in comfort eating because of its effect on mood and outlook.

Ask any therapist who uses food as a medium for improving health—naturopaths, homeopaths, acupuncturists. Wheat will always feature as the food presenting the most consistent problem to health because of overuse.

Of all the effects of foods on health and weight we've considered up to now, that of wheat is the most obvious as a demonstration of what a single food can do to your body/mind process, both in its short-term effects and its long-term consequences. Other carbohydrates can be a problem if overused, but none is so prevalent in our diet.

The wheat food that causes most problems is bread, because it is so readily available and so widely used. For many people it's a part of every meal they eat and of the snacks in between.

Naturally, I expect that the *Love Food . . . Lose Weight* diet will achieve marvels for you, but at the very least, if you take nothing else from reading this book, I advise you to change your habits with bread so you eat it no more than 1 in 5, preferably less. You'll notice the benefit very quickly.

Invariably, the responses I get from people who change their wheat habit are along the lines of: "I didn't believe it was possible for me to eat so little bread. Now I don't know how I ate so much" or "I feel uncomfortable every time I eat bread now." Notice they say they're still eating it. Well, *I* eat it—about once a week. I simply make sure that the day I eat it is a BFD (remember BFD—Best Food Day?). Late in the morning, one day a week, I go to a café where they have really good croissants and bread, great coffee, and a good view. I have my choice of bread spread thick with butter and jam, I drink my coffee, and I wile away an hour or so enjoying the view. I don't usually want to eat any more until the evening on those days because the bread fills me up—it bloats me a little. Later, for dinner, though not often, I might have pasta with my favorite sauce of tomatoes, peppers, olives, and garlic served with a crisp green salad.

The next day I'm three pounds heavier! I feel a bit lethargic and definitely a bit bigger around the middle. But these effects aren't a problem, because they've disappeared by the following day—and boy, have I enjoyed myself!

At all other times I avoid wheat as I'd avoid the plague—because I know if I eat it more than once a week, the effects will add up and initiate a domino effect in my system again. Every now and then I don't even go to the café for a couple of weeks, just to give myself a complete rest from wheat.

If, unusually, I want bread at any other time, I have whole rye bread. I stopped regularly wanting biscuits and cakes years ago, but on the odd occasions when I do want them, I go for oat biscuits. If I decide to have wheat, I'll have my favorites on my BFD.

My advice is to begin by avoiding wheat as much as possible for as long as you can by substituting some non-wheat alternatives on a 1 in 5 rotation. I know trying to imagine what to have for breakfast is a problem for quite a few people who have toast at the start of every day, but the menus you'll find later on will show how you can do it.

After you haven't eaten wheat for a while, try it again and see if it has any effect on you. Whether it does or not, whether you've avoided wheat for a long time or just for a few days, only eat wheat 1 in 5 at most.

The recipes and menus I provide in this book will show you how to combine wheat products into really enjoyable meals. At other times steer clear of wheat in all manufactured products. Remember, it's your Number One food enemy!

From Fat to Fit

The Master Plan which follows is a moderated and methodical way to get used to food combining and food rotation without running the risk of being overwhelmed by the confusion that often comes with trying something new for the first time. It also contains a variety of special techniques that will help you succeed with your diet and which, incidentally, will be useful to you in other ways if you choose to use them.

Ultimately what you achieve with *Love Food . . . Lose Weight* will depend on you, but right now it's time to take the first steps in improving your health and regaining control of your weight.

You can start looking forward to the wonderful feeling that

will come in a few days' and a few weeks' time, when you look back to today and become aware of changes and improvements you've brought about, to yourself, for yourself, by your own efforts.

CHAPTER

3

The Master Plan

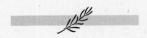

NICE AND EASY DOES IT!

Welcome to your first personal and direct experience of *Love Food . . . Lose Weight*! Over the next couple of weeks, I'd like to introduce you to some of the delights that this diet holds in store for you. It will be a benefit-packed fortnight which provides you with a strategy to help you through that initial learning period with the least effort and best results.

There's no need to feel apprehensive about committing yourself to a major change of lifestyle for two whole weeks. In fact, the Master Plan lasts for just *five days*—there are only five days of menus and food combinations to be concerned with—but I'd like you to *repeat* that five-day Master Plan three times . . . which actually comes to fifteen days, but you can take one day off for good behavior!

When you begin to learn something new, it takes time for you to become familiar with it. It takes time to master the basic skills and become proficient in them. So we're going to take things nice and easy—no fuss, no worrying about doing the wrong thing and, above all, no guilt or recriminations!

In these two weeks you'll experience the basics of food combining as they should be: a source of genuine pleasure from food and a simple and straightforward approach to lifelong health and weight control.

During this period you're going to learn *all* the essential knowledge you need to make the *Love Food . . . Lose Weight* diet work. The Master Plan provides a springboard that will enable you to further develop your diet at your own pace, using methods and skills I'll show you as we go along.

AN OVERVIEW OF THE MASTER PLAN

So that you're absolutely clear about what's involved in the Master Plan, I'd like to present you with a brief summary of what you will be doing over the next few days and weeks:

1. You'll devise an affirmation that you can use daily, in written and spoken form.
2. You'll create a mental picture with which to practice visualization for health and achievement.
3. You'll set and prioritize goals for your diet and your health.
4. You'll complete a Symptom Checklist before the Master Plan, and again when you have been on the diet for fourteen days.
5. You'll complete a five-day Diet Director to analyze your current diet.
6. You'll color in the Diet Director to highlight bad eating and food choices.
7. You'll set a starting date for the Master Plan.
8. You'll clear out your cupboards of bad food.
9. You'll become familiar with the Daily Menus and plan Five Days with the Menu Arranger.
10. You'll compose a shopping list of new, good foods.
11. You'll spend two delicious, quick and easy weeks on the Master Plan!

None of this is hard to do, and much of it is great fun—if you like questionnaires and quizzes, you'll have a ball!

WINNING THE MIND GAME

During the Master Plan you'll be using and benefiting from the natural laws that underpin everything you currently are and everything you are becoming.

In particular, you'll be using your mind as you've probably never used it before: as a tool for making conscious changes and improvements in yourself. To make something better happen, you only need to communicate to your inner self in convincing terms which you truly believe. This creates a new and better reality, first in what you believe about yourself, then, through the natural process of your body and mind working together, in your health, shape, and life.

You know now that your inner self-image has influenced the way you've been eating. To make a success of your new diet, it's essential that you improve the attitudes and beliefs that might be working against your health in the long term.

Your self-image is actually changing all the time, but mostly in small ways and then only reluctantly. The core substance of what you believe about yourself remains as it has been for years. And it will continue unchanged until you decide to focus your attention on it and remold it into how you want it to be.

Your inner self was produced from influences that acted within known principles. You can use those same principles to add new elements and create a self-image that will be working to *support* rather than *obstruct* your diet.

That's the mind game. Your self-image resists change if it can. To be successful at your new diet, to win through to a new level of health, you need to encourage your self-image to change in the best ways possible for you. And although your new diet is simultaneously creating the conditions which will make a change of your self-image easier, you also need to unite your new diet to new attitudes in a powerful alliance that will benefit you for the rest of your life.

First you need to recognize which beliefs may be holding you back from the health and shape you want. You probably already know but prefer not to acknowledge them, but when you concede what underlies your problem, you can convert harmful influences into powerfully constructive forces for helping you to become fitter and slimmer. You can make your negative attitudes into positive affirmations.

Making Affirmations Work for You

You made negative attitudes and beliefs into parts of your self-image in one of two ways. A single intense experience can imprint an event deep into your mind. You hold a memory of the event as well as the thoughts and feelings you experienced. You also retain memories of the consequences of that event, again with their associated thoughts and feelings.

The more usual way you acquired beliefs about yourself was by receiving and internalizing memories, thoughts, and feelings of the same messages repeated time and time again. When you were very young, you received a steady, repetitive diet of other people's opinions of you and what they thought you were capable of. Their opinions would have been the start of what you currently believe about yourself. You assumed certain attitudes about the world and how you saw yourself in it as a direct result of their recurring judgments.

However, neither intense single experiences from the past nor the repeated messages that became the truths in your inner self are likely to be the best basis for what you believe about yourself today. Even if they were correct at the time you acquired them, they are unlikely to be so now. Most of them, in any case, are based on the assumptions and opinions of others which, as you know, are very fallible.

You could try changing your unsuitable beliefs by therapy or in-depth analysis—or you can instead acquire new and more valuable attitudes *in the same ways* you picked up your old harmful ones.

That's the real beauty and power of using affirmations. This technique allows *you* to determine which new ideas you want to introduce into your self-image. In time the new ideas will naturally transform your current way of seeing and doing things. It's not a process of exorcising the old in favor of something new, but of expanding old notions so they can do more and do better.

Repeating the same message over and over again so that it becomes a part of you and therefore a basis for new behavior is called "making an affirmation." It is affirming a reality you believe is possible for you to experience. The practice of making affirmations is not new. Religions and faiths throughout the world have been doing it for centuries with prayers, chants, and mantras. Sports people, too, use repetition of positive phrases as a mind-management technique. In the first instance, repetition gets people in the frame of mind for spiritual advancement; in the second, repetition gets them in the frame of mind for physical achievement.

The sports person who repeats a positive message about their ability, over and over again, is building a mental foundation for what they want to do in physical reality. Just as repeating a certain physical exercise over and over makes a part of your body strong, repeating a belief over and over makes it a part of your mind. The sports person must start by accepting the possibility that they are capable of performing to the level they would like. Their mind/body process then takes over, and the *idea* within the positive repetition is turned into the *means* to make it happen.

Now, it's very important that you understand precisely *how* to use this powerful technique. Merely *thinking* a new idea—no matter how many times you do so—is *not* enough to make it real in your inner self. Thoughts and ideas already exist as normal chatter in the background of your mind; they run through your mind like sand through your fingers. The occasional "I can lose weight" or "I can be fitter and healthier" will be lost in an avalanche of the usual "I can't succeed at this" or "Nothing can change the way I look."

Here's the vital key to making affirmations really work for you: A *thought becomes significant only when it is acted upon.* The actions that anchor a new idea need not be extraordinary, just meaningful. If you underpin an idea by repeated meaningful actions, it becomes substantial enough in your mind to influence your reality. It is no longer a grain of sand among many, but becomes a seed that will grow into a new part of your reality.

Here are the techniques I recommend for creating and practicing affirmations. Once you've learned these techniques, you can use them in the future to transform all sorts of beliefs and attitudes, one at a time.

The more often you act meaningfully to substantiate an idea, the better the effect. The best way is to make your affirmation *systematically* and *consistently* for a specific period of time, so I suggest that you create and then practice your affirmation for an initial period of thirty days from the day you start the Master Plan.

The Right Affirmation for You

I've created four powerful affirmations for you to choose from. Each one addresses a different fundamental attitude which may be a problem. I'd like you to examine each affirmation and its explanation carefully and decide which is the most appropriate for you.

AFFIRMATION 1

Each new day I experience more and more peace in my life.

This affirmation addresses inappropriate anger. Reflect on your beliefs and attitudes and decide if you use anger in a suitable and life-enhancing way for your self and those around you. Determine whether anger plays a role which enables you to overcome problems in a reasonable way or if you are using it negatively and in circumstances where some other response or emotion is more valid. Evaluate the circumstances in which you become angry and the degree of anger you experience to see whether your anger is valid and useful to you or inhibiting to how you want to be. If your experience of anger is unsuitable, it will be affecting your body/mind system adversely and you should use Affirmation 1.

AFFIRMATION 2

Each new day I accept myself more and more for the unique person I am.

Affirmation 2 is designed to deal with your relationship with self-judgment. If you are excessively self-judgmental, feel you are not worthy of success or any of the benefits of life, this attitude will adversely affect your health and size through your body/mind process. Check out your level of self-judgment by observing how you react internally in different situations. Your body and your emotions will probably be involved in your responses. Are your assessments of your self honest, caring, and self-empowering or are they denigrating? Is the inner voice you hear one of disapproval, making you feel excessively guilty for small errors and shamed, or is it self-loving and helpful in doing better next time? If your self-judgment is overly critical, number 2 is the affirmation for you.

AFFIRMATION 3

Each new day I experience more and more the happiness I am capable of feeling.

The third affirmation is intended to resolve negative attitudes toward happiness. The questions you must ask yourself in connection with this affirmation are whether you feel happy most of the time or instead feel you cannot foresee being happy. Determine what your attitude toward happiness is. Is happiness something others experience but not you? Are your moments of happiness fleeting between long periods of non-feeling or sadness? If so, your affirmation is number 3.

AFFIRMATION 4

Each new day I express more and more of the courage of which I am capable.

Affirmation 4 relates to anxiety and fear when they are overwhelming attitudes which affect you through your body/mind process. Consider carefully whether you experience reasonable anxieties which keep you safe in appropriate ways during the day or if you feel an unsuitable level of fear in circumstances which are not really warranted for the adult you are. You might frequently experience feelings as if you were a child in situations over which you have no control. If fear/anxiety is not the helpful emotion, it should be for you. If your level of anxiety about your self and your life is excessive, then Affirmation 4 is the one for you.

If you feel that none of these is precisely appropriate to your needs, you can of course create your own affirmation, based on these themes. When devising an affirmation, encapsulate the most suitable new idea for you in words that you can accept as truly possible. The message must be powerful, meaningful, and positive. It also helps if it is simple and easy to recall from memory. Take your time creating your affirmation, rework it and reword it until you feel you can live with it, happily, for a long time. Then and only then should you begin to use it.

A Time and a Place for Affirmations

Choose a special time of day to make your affirmation. It should be at or around the same time each day, and at a time you know you can concentrate on what you are to do. Just before you go to sleep or first thing in the morning is best. Choose a special place to be when you make your affirmation. It should be somewhere you will be undisturbed and can relax for the ten minutes or so it will take. Play some gentle music and light a candle if you want to, as symbols to add emphasis to your intention—make making your affirmation an event!

Write Your Affirmation

When you write your affirmation down, it becomes meaningful. Write it daily and it becomes more meaningful. Write it several times in a day, and its consequences and potential are greatly magnified. Every day for thirty days, at your chosen time and place, write down your chosen affirmation ten times. If you use a large notepad, you will accumulate thirty sheets of paper with your affirmation written ten times on each. It's a good idea to number the sheets as you go to keep track. Remember, write your affirmation as a note to yourself, not to be shared. This is a personal process so keep your notepad private. After the thirtieth day, throw the lists away.

Speak Your Affirmation

Speaking a new idea aloud empowers it. Here a note of caution: speak your affirmation aloud *to yourself*. Sharing your affirmation with another introduces that person's opinion of you and invites them to express it. But it is not their belief about what you can do that matters here, it is yours. Speak your affirmation aloud ten times each day for thirty days. Try to stay attentive to what you are saying. Try to dissociate yourself from any doubt or inner chatter of disbelief. Make it real by choosing to believe it.

Protect Your Affirmation

During this thirty-day period, reinforce your affirmation by being aware of any negative thoughts that come to you during the day and construct a mental argument for supporting and believing your affirmation. At the same time, choose to act in ways that express how you expect to be rather than behaving in ways that strengthen your old attitudes. Use affirmations over these thirty days and your thought patterns will become more positive; the choices you make will begin to express your new attitude in increasingly obvious ways. Treat the few moments when you will actually be writing and speaking your affirmations as precious and inviolable. In this way your affirmation and all the benefits it brings will, like your new diet, become a powerful and sustaining part of your lifestyle.

Tips about Using Affirmations

You can strengthen your practice by giving yourself visual cues to remind you of your affirmation. Make a note of your chosen affirmation on a piece of colored card about the size of a credit card. Carry it with you in your diary, wallet, or purse so you will come across it frequently during the thirty days.

- Take a piece of card the same color as your credit card and cut it into pieces about an inch square. Stick the squares in strategic places where they won't be directly in your line of sight but will be in your peripheral vision. The edge of your bathroom or bedroom mirror, the corner of your car's rearview mirror, the corner of your computer screen or television, are good places. Remember, you shouldn't try to explain what you are doing to other people. Let them read *Love Food . . . Lose Weight* if they want to know. This is your personal process, and it's important you make it a private one.
- Associate your body with your affirmation. Make sure you hold yourself in the most confident posture you can imagine, as much as you can. Envisage the words of your affirmation, and as you inhale, imagine the words and their meaning circulating around your veins and arteries, becoming you.

- Whenever it comes to mind, repeat your affirmation a few times to yourself in your thoughts. In other words, keep it in mind as you go about your daily life. Certain things will remind you of it—don't let the moment pass but pause and recall your intention by saying the affirmation to yourself.

Visualization

There are other ways you can persuade your mind to accept a new idea and make it real for you.

Spend a little time observing skiers, race car drivers, and golfers, as just a few examples, and you'll often see them concentrating hard as they imagine the way they will race down the slope, or along the road, or how they will hit the ball. Some skiers, just before they compete, close their eyes and sway their bodies as they mentally ski the run. And before a race, many race car drivers let their eyes lose focus and flicker this way and that while in their minds they navigate around the track.

I remember an interview with Nigel Mansell, the world Formula One champion. He had astonished some baseball players in the United States because he had been able to hit nine out of ten fast balls launched at him by a pitching machine. Asked how he did it, he explained he just "saw" the balls coming at him bigger and more slowly. He used the same technique when racing, seeing in his mind's eye the corners coming toward him more slowly. He imagined he had plenty of time to hit the ball or steer the car. His body did the rest.

Such practices use the art of visualization to make real an ambition, goal, or intention. You, too, can use visualization to give substance to your goals and beliefs.

Your self-image, with all of its unhelpful beliefs and assumptions, quirky attitudes and inconsistencies, acts as an agenda for all the other functions of your body/mind.

You can use visualization to establish a new agenda, to set a new image and clarify what you expect of your body/mind processes. This is how you do it.

Once a day, at least, starting on the first day of your Master Plan, sit quietly for ten minutes or so, close your eyes, and visualize how you want to be. Visualize by imagining; create a mental picture of yourself, in every detail, that shows the person you really want to be. Picture your size and shape; imagine your demeanor and facial expression; visualize your movements, your manner of speaking. All are expressions of your inner self; envisage how you now prefer them to be.

As the days pass, add details to your original mental picture. Envisage yourself in the clothes you want to wear; in the activities you most enjoy and at which you are most talented. Especially imagine yourself eating well, enjoying the food, selecting appropriate foods for each meal and all the while becoming healthier, more vibrant, and more self-assured.

When practicing visualization, it's important to visualize the outcome you want without any judgment or opinion of how you might achieve it. In other words, see yourself as you would expect to be if you were as healthy and content as you can imagine. Visualize yourself as real: envisage the color and texture of your skin and hair; sense what emotions you would have in your mind; actually "see" and feel how you would be standing and breathing if you were as well and attractive as it is possible for you to be.

Allow your awareness to merge into your visualized self and experience what you would feel like to be so well. Practice feeling that way. Practice doesn't make perfect; practicing being perfect makes perfect.

- Visualization works best if you are physically relaxed and in a situation where, for ten minutes or so, there will be no distractions. You will know best where and at what time of day this is most feasible. Here's how to start: sit in a comfortable chair or lie on a bed or sofa, and close your eyes. Breathe deeply, in and out, ten times. With each breath out, imagine all your worries, aches, deadlines, shopping lists, and so on rushing out of your body, your mind, your life. Now create in your mind's eye the image of how you want to be. "See" what you intend your body and mind to create for you. Over the days and weeks ahead you can add details that will give meaning to what you want and expect from your body, your mind, and your life.

The purpose of these "mind game" techniques is to persuade your inner self that what you want is possible, beneficial, and safe. As a result of one or two successes in the mind game, you'll find yourself becoming increasingly discerning in your thought processes. Your thoughts and attitudes, then your words and actions, will take on a new significance for you, providing you with opportunities for change and improvement. You'll find yourself less willing to accept unhelpful and disabling thoughts, comments, and attitudes in yourself—and you'll now know you can change them.

I'm going to help you a little more to meet one or two goals you might have for your diet by suggesting you complete the Symptoms Checklist which follows before you start your Master Plan.

SYMPTOM CHECKLIST

The symptoms on the checklist that follows are indicators of disorder in your underlying health process. So much of your current health pattern has its origins in some time past. What we aim to do during the Master Plan is alter the course of this pattern so you will ultimately end up where you *want to be*, instead of where you're heading now.

Although it's impossible to work out precisely where the processes of your body and mind have become misdirected, your body/mind *knows instinctively*. Given the support it needs, it will automatically establish priorities and focus your resources for speedy improvement.

Symptoms take time to arise and even longer to become extreme. This diet brings about a gradual improvement in the underlying body/mind health process which can cause many of those symptoms to disappear spontaneously and others to reduce dramatically.

The approach is the same whatever the symptom. Even if you are particularly concerned about one or other of them, or even if you only want to deal with your weight problems, the Master Plan is still the first step to take toward improvement.

The checklist given here is intended to alert you to your present situation. By noting your symptoms, you gain the attention of your inner self and enlist all the support it can provide to overcome them. When you've been using the *Love Food . . . Lose Weight* diet for a while, you'll be able to return to this list to remind you where you were today, and to see how you've progressed.

To complete the checklist, first think about each symptom or problem marked in the left-hand column. If you don't suffer from the symptom, go straight on to the next. If, however, you do suffer from it, please indicate the degree of severity of the symptom, following the 1–8 scale at the top, by coloring in the boxes as appropriate. For example, if you suffer **Often** from **Allergies**, you might color the scale somewhere between the numbers 5 and 6, like this:

Allergies	now								

Make sure you shade the "Now" row; you're going to use the lower "Progress" row to monitor your progress later on. I suggest you use black or red to color or shade the Now row, so you can use a contrasting color when you repeat the list later. This is how your Allergy checklist might look after a month following *Love Food . . . Lose Weight*:

Allergies	now								
	progress								

If you mark a symptom **Extreme**, you may want to consult your doctor. *Love Food . . . Lose Weight* is compatible with medical treatment and alternative therapies, and will not affect or be affected by treatments you need. You should discuss what you are doing with your health professional, especially if you are under medical supervision.

SYMPTOM CHECKLIST

		None or Never		Mild or Sometimes		Moderate or Often		Extreme or Always	
		1	2	3	4	5	6	7	8
Abdominal distension	now								
	progress								
Acne	now								
	progress								
Allergies	now								
	progress								

SYMPTOM CHECKLIST

		None or Never		Mild or Sometimes		Moderate or Often		Extreme or Always	
		1	2	3	4	5	6	7	8
Anal itching/	now								
hemorrhoids	progress								
Arthritis	now								
	progress								
Asthma	now								
	progress								
Bags under	now								
eyes	progress								
Bloating	now								
	progress								
Blood	now								
pressure	progress								
Body odor	now								
	progress								
Burping	now								
	progress								
Cellulite	now								
	progress								
Cholesterol	now								
	progress								
Clarity of	now								
thought	progress								
Cold	now								
extremities	progress								

SYMPTOM CHECKLIST

		None or Never		Mild or Sometimes		Moderate or Often		Extreme or Always	
		1	2	3	4	5	6	7	8
Cold sores	now								
	progress								
Cold sweats	now								
	progress								
Colon health	now								
	progress								
Complexion	now								
problems	progress								
Confidence	now								
problems	progress								
Duodenal	now								
ulcer	progress								
Eczema	now								
	progress								
Eyes sensitive	now								
to light	progress								
Fatigue	now								
	progress								
Fingernail	now								
problems	progress								
Flatulence	now								
	progress								
Fluid	now								
retention	progress								

SYMPTOM CHECKLIST

		None or Never		Mild or Sometimes		Moderate or Often		Extreme or Always	
		1	2	3	4	5	6	7	8
Food cravings	now								
	progress								
Food intolerance	now								
	progress								
Frequent colds	now								
	progress								
Gallbladder problems	now								
	progress								
Hair condition problems	now								
	progress								
Hay fever	now								
	progress								
Headaches	now								
	progress								
Hunger pangs	now								
	progress								
Hyperactivity	now								
	progress								
Hyperglycemia	now								
	progress								
Hypoglycemia	now								
	progress								
Indigestion	now								
	progress								

SYMPTOM CHECKLIST

		None or Never		Mild or Sometimes		Moderate or Often		Extreme or Always	
		1	2	3	4	5	6	7	8
Insomnia	now								
	progress								
Irritability	now								
	progress								
Joint pain	now								
	progress								
Joint swelling	now								
	progress								
Lack of appetite	now								
	progress								
Lack of energy	now								
	progress								
Libido problems	now								
	progress								
Low back pain	now								
	progress								
Melancholy/ depression	now								
	progress								
Migraines	now								
	progress								
Mood swings	now								
	progress								
Mouth ulcers	now								
	progress								

SYMPTOM CHECKLIST

		None or Never		Mild or Sometimes		Moderate or Often		Extreme or Always	
		1	2	3	4	5	6	7	8
Muscle aches	now								
	progress								
Muscle cramps	now								
	progress								
Muscle tension	now								
	progress								
Muscle tone problems	now								
	progress								
Nausea	now								
	progress								
Neck and shoulder pain	now								
	progress								
Nervousness	now								
	progress								
Pallor	now								
	progress								
Peptic ulcer	now								
	progress								
Persistent thirst	now								
	progress								
PMS	now								
	progress								
Psoriasis	now								
	progress								

SYMPTOM CHECKLIST

		None or Never		Mild or Sometimes		Moderate or Often		Extreme or Always	
		1	2	3	4	5	6	7	8
Psychological disorders	now								
	progress								
Puffy eyes	now								
	progress								
Self-esteem problems	now								
	progress								
Sensitivity to cold	now								
	progress								
Sinus conditions	now								
	progress								
Size changes	now								
	progress								
Skin quality problems	now								
	progress								
Sleep problems	now								
	progress								
Stress	now								
	progress								
Temperament problems	now								
	progress								
Tinnitus	now								
	progress								
Weight gain	now								
	progress								

SYMPTOM CHECKLIST

		None or Never		Mild or Sometimes		Moderate or Often		Extreme or Always	
		1	2	3	4	5	6	7	8
Weight loss	now								
	progress								
Yeast	now								
imbalance	progress								

Color Your Diet!

You're going to find this quite an eye-opener.

Until you know what the problem areas in your diet are, it's hard to start correcting them. Unfortunately, we constantly deceive ourselves about the type, quantity, and quality of the food we eat . . . you know what I mean! So here is a quick and conclusive way to identify the problem areas in your present eating pattern and bring them right to your attention—by color! Using the following Five-Day Eating Record, write down everything you had to eat or drink yesterday and today. Do the same for the next three days. When the form is complete, you can go through it identifying and highlighting any appearance of the Five Eating Patterns described below. Then you'll instantly see just how good or bad your diet has become. You'll also be able to pinpoint which bad eating habits you're going to address with the Master Plan.

FIVE-DAY EATING RECORD

	YESTERDAY	TODAY	DAY 3	DAY 4	DAY 5
Midnight–7:00 am					
Breakfast 7:00 am–10:00 am					

FIVE-DAY EATING RECORD

	YESTERDAY	TODAY	DAY 3	DAY 4	DAY 5
10:00 am–Noon					
Lunch Noon–3:00 pm					
3:00 pm–6:00 pm					
Dinner 6:00 pm–10:00 pm					
10:00 pm–Midnight					

Now, choose five different-colored pens or highlighters. Look at the table which follows and choose one color to represent each of the Five Eating Patterns, then mark that color in the Color Code box to show what it means.

EATING PATTERN   YOUR COLOR CODE

EATING PATTERN	YOUR COLOR CODE
1. Meals in which Protein foods have been mixed with Carbohydrate foods. Or meals containing either food eaten within four hours of the other.	
2. Meals which contain wheat, oats, barley, or rye.	
3. Meals containing cheese, ice cream, or chocolate.	
4. Drinks or foods containing caffeine—coffee, tea, cola, or chocolate.	
5. Foods you eat often—i.e. every day or nearly daily—except fresh fruits and Mix With Any vegetables or salads.	

Next, you must check through the five-day record of your food intake and highlight—in the appropriate colors—any of the above five eating patterns you find. Be ruthless! The more color you see on the food record, the more problems there are in your diet. And the more often a color appears, the more often you're repeating the same problem. This is a graphic and unequivocal way to identify unhelpful eating patterns so that you can begin to do something about them. Let's look at each one in turn.

Problem 1. Bad Combining

The first problem, bad combining, is simple to address. You'll be food combining correctly with the Master Plan just by following the menus as they are, or by using the Five-Day Menu Arranger.

Problem 2. Overuse of Cereals

Of the cereals listed in the second Eating Pattern, I've already discussed wheat at length (see page 50). Most of the time you use this color, it will probably indicate wheat, but all of the cereals listed in this eating pattern contain gluten—and sometimes it is gluten, not simply wheat, that is the problem. In the Master Plan you're going to eat wheat 1 in 5, but I suggest you treat oats, barley, and rye as if they were wheat, too. In other words, don't reduce your wheat intake to 1 in 5 but then replace it with a daily diet of oats or barley or rye. Treat these foods as a group that shouldn't be eaten more than 1 in 5.

Problem 3. Cow's-Milk Foods

Cheese, ice cream, and chocolate are high-fat cow's dairy foods. Products with concentrated cow's milk often cause problems, so on the Master Plan cow's dairy products should form a group that should be eaten no more than 1 in 5.

Problem 4. Caffeine

Caffeine is a powerful drug. It affects your mind and various organs in your body. The more you use it, the more you'll need. You won't be doing anything about caffeine during the Master Plan fortnight, but you should still become aware of how much you are using it and which products and meals contain it.

It took me well over a year before I finally had to recognize the fact that caffeine was the only habit food I was using that I hadn't challenged, though I was trying to limit chocolate and sugar overuse. Making caffeine a 1 in 5 completely changed my ability to sustain energy levels and optimism, as it has for many others I've known. By changing my use of caffeine, my chocolate and sugar overuse disappeared. I'll show you how to reduce and control your intake a little later in this book—withdrawal from caffeine needs planning.

Problem 5. Habitual Foods

Last but not least are the foods you eat habitually. This usually means daily or nearly daily. Don't worry about fresh fruit, vegetables, or salads—the more you eat of these the better! Although the Master Plan will take care of most of your habit foods with the built-in food-rotation strategy, you should know which foods you may be using as a "crutch" (they commonly include milk, salty foods including chips, peanuts, and soy sauce, or very sweet foods including dry fruits) because you'll want to challenge them after you've been on this diet for a while.

SUCCESS IS ALL A MATTER OF TIMING

Today, set a special starting date for your Master Plan. This can be a powerful device for making sure you succeed. By setting a date for starting a little in the future, you can generate excitement, enthusiasm, expectation, and commitment. These feelings are resources that are far more useful to you than the short-lived zeal that comes with an impulsive decision to jump into a diet.

Make your choice of this date with care and consideration. Set it far enough ahead to give you time to make arrangements and prepare yourself. But not so far ahead that you lose momentum.

Get out a calendar or your diary. Choose a day that's convenient, preferably not more than a week away but no sooner than three days. If there is some special significance that attracts you to one day over others, choose that day. Now "red star" your chosen starting day in your diary or calendar. In fact, write it here:

I BEGIN MY LOVE FOOD . . . LOSE WEIGHT MASTER PLAN ON:

Date: _____

Here's a list of what you should do before you start the Master Plan. Check off each item as you complete it.

THE FINAL COUNTDOWN

Days to go	Do this	Check when complete
5	Complete initial Symptom Checklist (page 66)	
	Start filling in the form to Color Your Diet (page 73)	
	Choose the colors for your diet (page 74)	
4	Choose your affirmation (page 59)	
3	Make sure you've set your Starting Date (above)	
	Eat up your garbage (page 78)	
	Complete first Five-Day Menu Arranger (page 90)	
2	Get pad and pencil for affirmations	
	Produce First Shopping List and restock with helpful foods (page 92)	
1	Finish coloring your diet (pages 73–75)	
0	GO! Start Your Master Plan	
	Start thirty days of written and spoken affirmations	

Now you're ready to organize the practical details that will make your diet so easy and natural.

WAIST DISPOSAL

One of the most amusing situations I encounter with wealthy clients often happens when I'm helping them—at their invitation—plan their meals. I usually nose around in their refrigerators and cupboards to see what they have there.

I'm sure I could write a book from those experiences alone—*Refrigerators of the Rich and Famous*. Almost invariably, among the caviar and asparagus, I've found little pots of food left over from previous meals . . . "Just in case I feel peckish" or "So it won't go to waste." Yes, even the wealthy don't like waste!

I remember on one occasion lining up about a dozen plastic pots with lids—each pot no bigger than a small cup. "That's about twenty cents worth of potato," I called out. "Fifteen cents worth of cold chicken" (not enough for a meal, but "enough to nibble at") "and ten cents worth of sweet corn." The list went on and on, and each item was something that should be eaten on the 1 in 5 rotation, so shouldn't be kept for another day anyway!

It just isn't worth hanging onto odd scraps of food left over from a meal. Even when they aren't foods that should be rotated, there's going to be little goodness left in them after they've been prepared, cooked, and stored. Get into the habit from now on of throwing away what you have left after a meal. Each meal will then be freshly prepared and freshly considered in combining and rotating terms.

In the cupboard another story unfolds. Boxes and cans of wonderful soups and processed foods from the most exclusive shops . . . each one a food combiner's nightmare. My point is, having some kinds of foods around will *hinder* your success. You should clear your cupboards of them.

Now, please stay calm: just because you're getting them out of your cupboard and out of everyday reach doesn't mean you'll never be able to eat them again. It just means you'll have to make an effort to get them—and that gives you the opportunity to decide if you *really* want them.

At times you'll want to reach into your cupboard for something easy. If that happens when you're hungry and tired and what you take out doesn't fit the new rules—bang goes your diet. And bang goes a little of the new reality you're trying to establish, because you'll have *undermined* your goal of eating correctly. You can't say to yourself that from now on, you're going to eat correctly combined meals if all you've got in your cupboard is bread and cheese. When you want a quick and properly combined meal, you simply won't have what you need. In that moment your Master Plan can fly out the window, and all your good intentions can go with it.

Now—before your official starting date—is the time to sort through any foods you have that won't fit into your new diet. Items like processed and prepared foods that are badly combined. Items like bread and snacks made from wheat. Also any other 1 in 5 foods such as cheese, potatoes, or chocolate. And especially items that have become a favorite part of your diet, because that means they are part of your eating problem. Give them away, feed them to the dog, eat them up, throw them out—anything, but get them out of your cupboard before you begin.

- To avoid unnecessary waste in future, use 1 in 5 foods as the main item in a meal and buy it the day you intend to use it. That way you can make it a Best Food Day and enjoy the best quality of your favorite 1 in 5 food.
- If there's too much to throw out, freeze it. Having to thaw food out gives you time to think about whether you really want to eat it.

FOURTEEN DAYS OF MENU INSPIRATIONS

Most people's minds go completely blank when they're confronted with a change of diet. Invariably the question uppermost in their minds is: "But what *can* I eat?" The human mind can take a very narrow view when it feels threatened!

With the Master Plan you won't have any problems. For fourteen days you simply make your daily choices for each meal from the menus I've created for you. You'll automatically be following the rules of combining and rotating *without the need to worry about what you can and cannot eat*. You'll also be learning just how enjoyable healthy eating can be. Here's what to do.

Remember, you're going to be repeating a fundamental five-day eating plan three times over the next two weeks. This means that there are only *five* days of menus and food combinations to be bothered with—which makes it easy on you. However, just in case some people start to feel a little restricted on a five-day eating plan, I've given you a *choice of menus* for each day. So for five days you'll have two menus to choose from, Option A and Option B. Each Daily Menu Option gives you a suggestion for breakfast, lunch, and dinner. All you have to do to stay within the healthy eating rules is pick Option A or Option B each day and follow the menus shown. When you reach Day Five, just return to Day One and start going through the days again. Continue choosing Option A or Option B from Day One to Day Five until you have completed fourteen days of healthy eating. Easy!

Even if you take the simplest way and choose Option A on each of your first five days and Option B for each of the second five days, you'll have had different meals for ten of the fourteen days.

The Daily Menus from the Master Plan show you just one way in which it's possible to distribute proteins and carbohydrates over five days, within the combining and rotating rules. It's an easy way to get started. In due course you'll be able to make your own choices without any problem, but for now, simply eat the meals as shown and you'll be eating well without having to suffer dieters' confusion.

You may be wondering if you should limit the amount of food you eat. After all, you're supposed to be on a diet, aren't you—and dieting is supposed to hurt! Well, with *Love Food . . . Lose Weight*, the quantity of food you eat is not very significant. Your main focus should be on keeping to the rules of combining and rotating foods. Remember, the main purpose of this diet is to stop your body from creating more toxicity than it can cope with. When you stop producing toxins by eating correctly, your body will be able to restore itself to health by its own natural processes. Don't eat more than you would normally, but you needn't go out of your way to eat less at the moment.

For your health and your weight remember these basic tips:

Tip One: Try to simplify your diet as much as possible. You will digest your meals more easily and will benefit more rapidly from simple meals. In fact, as your system responds to the diet, you'll find your desire for complicated meals and rich food will naturally diminish in favor of simpler meals. You'll be able to taste and enjoy what you are eating more. You won't need elaborate sauces, and suddenly too many proteins or carbohydrates in a meal will not suit you.

Tip Two: Avoid using too many proteins or carbohydrates each day. Mixing several proteins or carbohydrates in a meal makes rotation more difficult. You'll notice each meal on your Master Plan rarely uses more than one protein or carbohydrate. In any case, you don't want to end up one day hunting around desperately for something you haven't already eaten in the previous four.

Tip Three: It is not compulsory to eat everything that's shown for each meal. The menus have been devised to provide you healthy multi-course meals to show you what is possible. For instance, the menus often suggest light starters of soup or salad, for these will ensure you won't need large portions of the main courses or desserts. But if you usually eat only one or two courses, please continue to do that now, choosing from the courses shown here.

Tip Four: If you are especially interested in losing weight, it's sensible not to overeat. Eat the same amount as you usually do, or perhaps a little less, but stay firmly on track with your combining and rotating by choosing what you eat from the Daily Menu Options available. Try to eat only moderate amounts of proteins or carbohydrates and plenty of vegetables and salads.

Tip Five: You can help your weight control even more if you keep your intake of fats and oils to a minimum and especially avoid putting them with carbohydrates. Try to avoid those Daily Menu Options with higher fat contents, don't use fatty spreads such as butter or margarine on bread or crackers, and leave the skin off poultry and meat proteins.

Tip Six: During the Master Plan you can be reducing your cow's dairy intake (including concentrated dairy products) and your saturated fat intake considerably. Just choose the Options which don't feature these types of food and start to use unsaturated oils in your cooking and salad dressings, preferably nut and vegetable oils that haven't been refined— because they are easier to digest. Milk is an obvious cow's dairy product many people overuse, so take it in small amounts only for the moment, with a mind to challenging it at some time in the future.

ADVICE FOR VEGETARIANS

Love Food . . . Lose Weight is entirely compatible with vegetarian eating. Indeed, it improves the average vegetarian diet and makes it even more healthy and weight-friendly.

A common problem for veggies is overuse of some foods. They often replace animal-protein foods with a limited selection of carbohydrates, which results in their overuse—particularly of wheat, potatoes, rice, and beans. The consequences are far from the good diet most vegetarians aim for, so weight and health can both suffer.

Poor combining is not a great problem for vegetarians, although it can occur when nuts, seeds, or soy are mixed with carbohydrates in a meal. Another problem is mixing too many main carbohydrates or proteins together in the same meal, even if proteins and carbohydrates are being properly separated. A complicated meal which contains rice, potatoes, and beans would be quite common, and can easily be simplified to great benefit.

Apply the food-combining and food-rotation rules to vegetarian foods, and you'll have the best of both worlds. If you separate nonanimal proteins (like nuts and soy) from your carbohydrates and vary them to 1 in 5, you'll get wonderful results. The best thing to do is to feature just one of these foods in each meal and really enjoy as many vegetable or salad foods as you can put with it.

Vegetables can be stir-fried, curried, roasted, broiled, or chopped, and made into salads, and all can be delicious when accompanied by a non-animal protein or one of the carbohydrates.

The following is an example of how to vary the main non-animal proteins and carbohydrates to achieve 1 in 5 rotation. There are many suggestions and much advice that's relevant for vegetarians in the

Daily Menus. You'll find a few veggie recipes for you in the Master Plan, and I'm sure you can think of many other delicious ways to combine your foods correctly into wonderful meals.

VEGETARIAN FIVE-DAY FOOD ARRANGER
P = Protein Foods, C = Carbohydrate Foods

	Day 1	Day 2	Day 3	Day 4	Day 5
Fruit any day (fresh, stewed, or juiced) - see advice on page 41					
Breakfast (choose from)	C Gluten grain (wheat, oats, or rye)	P Yogurt (cow's milk)	C Corn cereal	P Yogurt (sheep's or goat's milk)	C Rice cereal
Lunch or Dinner (choose from)	P Soy C Gluten grain (wheat, oats, or rye)	P Walnuts Cashews C Millet and Beans	P Pine nuts Almonds C Corn	P Pumpkin seeds C Potatoes	P Hazelnuts Sunflower seeds C Rice Buckwheat

Your options are even more varied if you eat cheese and eggs in your vegetarian diet. You simply need to be careful that you don't combine them with carbohydrates, since they are both proteins. In chapter 6 are some delicious recipes with eggs and cheese.

MASTER PLAN DAILY MENUS

Now let's have a look at the Daily Menus, the recipes for which appear in chapter 6. Study the Menus, then use the Five-Day Menu Arranger on page 90 to help you set out the Options you will eat for the first five days of your own Master Plan. The recipes and an ingredients checklist for all the following menus are given in chapter 6.

MASTER PLAN DAILY MENU—DAY 1

	Option A	Option B
Breakfast	Fresh fruits (F) Your choice of at least three different varieties	Gluten grains (C) oat porridge or rye toast or crackers
Morning Snacks	Your choice, but see the advice on page 89	
Lunch	Mushroom soup (M/A) Couscous and mixed vegetables with piquant sauce (C) Mint ice (C)	Spinach and pea soup (M/A) Salmon with vegetables and spinach sauce (P) Green salad with dessert vinaigrette (M/A)
Afternoon Snacks	Your choice, but see the advice on page 89	
Dinner	Smoked salmon salad (P) Turkey cutlets with ribbon vegetables and herb sauce (P) Tomato salad with dessert vinaigrette (M/A)	Avocado with tomato, onion, and basil salsa (M/A) Pasta with chilies and mixed sweet peppers (C) White wine ice (C)
Your 1 in 5 Foods	Gluten grain: Wheat (couscous) Salmon Turkey	Gluten grain: Oats or rye Wheat (pasta) Salmon

MASTER PLAN DAILY MENU—DAY 2

	Option A	Option B
Breakfast	Fresh fruits (F) Your choice of at least three different varieties	Fresh fruits (F) Your choice of at least three different varieties
Morning Snacks	Your choice, but see the advice on page 89	
Lunch	Creamy onion soup (M/A) Warm salad of mixed mushrooms (M/A) Cheese and walnuts with crudités (P)	Creamy celery soup (M/A) Steak and mixed salad (P) Cheese and crudités with onion chutney (P)
Afternoon Snacks	Your choice, but see the advice on page 89	
Dinner	Cauliflower cheese soup (P) Cashews and stir-fry vegetables (P) Green salad with dessert vinaigrette (M/A)	Herby green salad (M/A) Roast fish with oven-cooked ratatouille (P) Yogurt with chopped Brazil nuts (P)
Your 1 in 5 Foods	Cheese (cow's milk) Walnuts Cashews	Cow's milk, cheese, and yogurt Beef (steak) Fish Brazil nuts

MASTER PLAN DAILY MENU—DAY 3

	Option A	Option B
Breakfast	Stewed fruits (F) Your choice of dried fruits stewed with honey and orange peel	Corn cereal with half-and-half and water (C) or Yogurt with stewed fruit (P)
Morning Snacks	Your choice, but see the advice on page 89	
Lunch	Green salad (M/A) Polenta with Mediterranean-style vegetables and herb tomato sauce (C) Chocolate sorbet (C)	Mushroom soup (M/A) Roasted, herbed vegetables, with pine nuts and tomatoes (P) Green salad with dessert vinaigrette (M/A)
Afternoon Snacks	Your choice, but see the advice on page 89	
Dinner	Pumpkin soup (M/A) Chicken kebabs with herbed ribbon vegetables and purée of celery root (P) Green salad with dessert vinaigrette (M/A)	Herby green salad (M/A) Chicken breast stuffed with spicy vegetables on spinach with purée of carrot (P) Yogurt with chopped almonds (P)
Your 1 in 5 Foods	Corn (polenta) Chocolate Chicken	Corn (cereal) Pine nuts Chicken Almonds Yogurt

MASTER PLAN DAILY MENU—DAY 4

	Option A	Option B
Breakfast	Ham and egg with tomatoes and mushrooms (P)	Fresh fruits (F) Your choice of at least three different varieties
Morning Snacks	Your choice, but see the advice on page 89	
Lunch	Creamy onion soup (M/A) Potatoes Sicilian-style with green salad (C) Mint ice (C)	Bacon and avocado salad (P) Vegetable frittata with oven-cooked ratatouille (P) Green salad with dessert vinaigrette (M/A)
Afternoon Snacks	Your choice, but see the advice on page 89	
Dinner	Mushroom soup (M/A) Quick roast pork BBQ-style, with stir-fry vegetables (P) Green salad with dessert vinaigrette (M/A)	Spinach and pea soup (M/A) Boulangère potatoes with mixed salad (C) White wine ice (C)
Your 1 in 5 Foods	Pork (ham) Eggs Potatoes	Pork (bacon) Eggs (frittata) Potatoes

MASTER PLAN DAILY MENU—DAY 5

	Option A	Option B
Breakfast	Stewed fruits (F) Your choice of dried fruits stewed with honey and orange peel	Rice breakfast cereal with half-and-half and water or Rice Dream (C)
Morning Snacks	Your choice, but see the advice below	
Lunch	Avocado soup (M/A) Hot and sour fish on vegetable noodles (P) Green salad with dessert vinaigrette (M/A)	(no starter) Roast cod on shell-fish soup with herby green salad (P) Yogurt and chopped hazelnuts (P)
Afternoon Snacks	Your choice, but see the advice below	
Dinner	Hummus with crudités (C) Risotto of mixed mushrooms (C) Mint ice (C)	Mixed salad with olives (M/A) Lamb roasted Greek-style, with oven-cooked ratatouille (P) Goat's and sheep's cheeses with crudité (P)
Your 1 in 5 Foods	Lamb (liver) Chickpeas (hummus) Rice (risotto) Fish (sea bass, monkfish)	Rice cereal Cod Shellfish Hazelnuts Cheese (goat and sheep) Lamb Yogurt (sheep)

The Five-Day Menu Arranger (see next page) enables you to record your choice of Options for periods of five days at a time. Simply jot down your menu Options (A or B) under the appropriate Day and next to the Meal time of day. The 1 in 5 foods you can use each day are listed at the bottom of the Daily Menus. To teach yourself to keep track of them, simply make a note of the ones you actually choose to eat in the Summary below each day on the Menu Arranger.

During the Master Plan fortnight, I recommend you complete a Menu Arranger every five days and stick to it. If you prefer to rearrange the Options to suit yourself or try out other recipes, use the same blank form but write a brief description of the meals you plan to eat. If you don't know what you are going to eat at a meal—because you are eating at a restaurant, for example—write it down in the space *after* you've eaten. Recording what you ate is a good way to stay focused on your diet in that first important period.

Arrange as many Five-Day Menus as you need until you are *completely comfortable* with combining and rotating, and can make good choices spontaneously, or until you no longer need the help they will give you to stay on track.

COPING WITH SNACK ATTACKS

One last thing before we move on: snacks aren't compulsory! I've left room for snacks on the Menu Arranger so you can jot them down *if* you eat them. Doing this will help you by making you think twice before you snack, and show you just what you are eating, if you have to write them down each time. However, if you make sure you eat sufficiently at each planned meal, especially at breakfast, you'll find you won't need to snack so much—if at all. It's a false economy of effort to eat too little food at a meal, then find you have to surrender to a snack attack later during the day. Frankly, this—more than almost anything else—risks jeopardizing your proper food combining and rotation.

If you do have a serious snack attack, use the *ten minute time-out*. Cravings have been shown to last only a short time, and if they are not accommodated right away they can pass harmlessly by. If you have a sudden need for a snack, just say to yourself, "Time-out. In ten minutes if I still want a snack I'll have it," and get on with what you were

YOUR FIVE-DAY MENU ARRANGER

	KW	DAY 1	DAY 2	DAY 3	DAY 4	DAY 5
Breakfast						
Snacks						
Lunch						
Snacks						
Dinner						
Snacks						
Summary 1 in 5 Foods Used						

doing—or find something to do to take your attention elsewhere. Odds are, you'll forget you even had a snack attack.

However, we all have a need to indulge in treats at times or perhaps succumb to a craving, so when you do yield to temptation, try to make your snacks healthy Mix With Any foods such as crudités. If you can't manage this, at least try to have easy-to-digest foods such as fruit or yogurt which can be eaten up to an hour before other types of foods without compromising your diet. Otherwise, try to choose something which is compatible with the meal nearest to which the snack is being eaten. For example, if your nearest meal was a carbohydrate, have a carbohydrate snack such as oatcakes or potato chips. If the nearest is to be a protein, choose nuts—but not peanuts, which are carbohydrates.

Be aware that a craving or strong desire for a particular snack may be because of a need for some food to which you are addicted, or which is part of a sensitivity problem. Salty snacks such as salted nuts and chips, sugar-rich snacks such as confectionery and sweets, wheat snacks such as biscuits and crackers, high-fat snacks such as ice cream, cheese, and fried foods, and caffeine-rich snacks including chocolate are all prime suspects here.

In the short term, try to substitute more healthy alternatives for these cravings until you can have the food you need in a main meal. After being on this diet a while, you should find your snack cravings diminish until your food needs are taken care of by your regular meals.

YOUR FIRST SHOPPING LIST

A couple of days before your starting date, provide yourself with a stockpile of useful foods from which to prepare delicious, quick, and easy meals that fit your new eating pattern.

Restocking your pantry is an *investment*. It's part of the preparation that will mean the difference between succeeding and progressing to further benefits—or failing and reinforcing a "I-can't-get-healthier-or-slimmer" reality.

It's important your stock foods are ones you *like*! Also, make sure that what you keep readily available doesn't tempt you to combine badly, or to eat 1 in 5 foods more often than you should. If you refer to your color-coded diet analysis (see page 74), you will see which bad foods you have been using routinely. Those are the foods to *avoid having around you now*.

Restocking provides an opportunity for you to include more variety in your diet and to experiment with tastes and textures that will reawaken your pleasure in food. I use restocking as a chance to gather together a variety of flavorings (most are Mix With Any foods) that I can use freely to make every meal an enjoyable experience.

Here's a sample First Shopping List of foods to get you started. There are fresh foods, unusual delicacies to add that extra something to a meal, and a few cans for emergencies. The only other items you might need are those for your first few meals. Add those items when you've decided what your first meals on the Master Plan will be (see Five-Day Menu Arranger, page 90).

FIRST SHOPPING LIST

Check items you need to buy   y/c = your choice

- ❑ Anchovies (can)
- ❑ Apricots (dried)
- ❑ Baked beans (can)
- ❑ Balsamic vinegar
- ❑ Black pepper
- ❑ Broccoli
- ❑ Butter
- ❑ Capers
- ❑ Carrots
- ❑ Cauliflower
- ❑ Chicory
- ❑ Coffee
- ❑ Cream (single)
- ❑ Cucumber
- ❑ Dried spices (y/c)
- ❑ Fruit juice (y/c)
- ❑ Fruits (fresh) (y/c)
- ❑ Green beans
- ❑ Herbs (fresh) (y/c)
- ❑ Herbs (dried) (y/c)
- ❑ Leeks
- ❑ Lettuce (y/c)

- ❑ Milk
- ❑ Mustard
- ❑ Olive oil
- ❑ Olives
- ❑ Peas (frozen)
- ❑ Pine kernels
- ❑ Prunes (can or dry)
- ❑ Rice
- ❑ Rye crispbread
- ❑ Salad onions
- ❑ Sea salt
- ❑ Sesame oil (toasted)
- ❑ Spinach (frozen)
- ❑ Tabasco
- ❑ Tea
- ❑ Tomatoes (fresh)
- ❑ Tomatoes (can)
- ❑ Tuna fish (can)
- ❑ Vegetable juice
- ❑ Wine
- ❑ Wine or cider vinegar
- ❑ Zucchini

During the Master Plan, your meals are planned for you. For any day you can look at the Daily Menu sheets (page 84) and choose what you'd like to eat from the options available. The items you'll need for your shopping list are shown with the recipes (see page 196) for each option. Just add them to your shopping list. What could be easier?

A FEW WORDS OF ADVICE

Love Food . . . Lose Weight is one of the easiest "diets" you've ever encountered. If you're anything like my clients, you'll soon find the basic principles become an instinctive part of your way of life . . . which is exactly how it should be! Of course, *any* change of food can create some initial questions in people's minds, so here are answers to the most frequent queries.

Breakfast can be a problem for people who are just starting out. Many take little time or trouble over it, and they usually eat the same thing every day: something like toast or breakfast cereals, tea or coffee, maybe fruit juice and perhaps a piece of fruit. That or nothing at all.

Findings have suggested that just fruit is the best breakfast because the human digestive system has a biological rhythm that makes it poor at digesting anything but fruit before midday. There may be some truth in that. After many years of eating this diet, I find my breakfasts have gradually changed until now I simply prefer to eat a variety of fruits for breakfast each morning.

Some experts cite the soporific effects of cereals as reason not to eat carbohydrates on rising; others speak of the stimulating effects of proteins and suggest they would be good to eat first thing in the day. The fact is, individual requirements and the effects of prolonged poor eating have produced a whole variety of different needs. Some people find they want carbohydrates early in the day; others want proteins, regardless of how their digestion is supposed to work or maybe because of the effects proteins have on their brain. So what should you do?

Your Daily Menus give you various breakfast Options on most days. **Fruit** is easy to digest and has several particular advantages as a breakfast, so it appears at least once every day as an Option. Fruit helps to keep your bowel moving and your colon healthy. Fruit is high in water and low in calories, so it assists with the removal of toxins you'll be cleansing on your Master Plan, and helps you lose weight. It's a good idea to have fruit breakfasts as often as you can, *but you don't have to force yourself*. Eat other foods occasionally as long as they are properly combined and rotated, and eventually you'll find your body will indicate what it needs most.

Milk often features heavily at breakfast, both on cereals and in drinks. Under the food-combining rule milk combines badly with cereals, which are carbohydrates. In any case, milk is one of those foods that's often overused. In the Master Plan, my advice is to reduce your intake of milk to small amounts only, and to use alternatives when possible. But don't worry about making it 1 in 5 unless you know you have a problem with it.

If you want something to put on breakfast **cereals** you can use light cream diluted at least half and half with water. When making oatmeal, use water with a little cream if you like, but of course you must be careful with cream—which is a high-fat food—if you want to lose weight.

There is a nondairy milk product in health food stores called Rice Dream. It's made from rice, as you'd imagine, and therefore combines well with cereals. In your Daily Menus I've suggested you use it only on rice cereals to make sure rice is used only 1 in 5—but you could use it occasionally on other cereals.

Small amounts of milk in tea or coffee won't cause a problem for most people, but even then you could use **soy milk** or half-and-half and water. Note that soy milk won't combine with cereals.

After you've been on the diet for a while you may want to challenge your use of cow's-milk products to find out if they are a problem for you. Each of the three *Love Food . . . Lose Weight* Strategies in chapter 4 shows how to gradually reduce certain problem foods. You can use the same technique to gradually reduce your cow's dairy foods intake until you can remove them entirely for a while. After they've been out of your diet for ten days or so, you'll have a good sense of what effect they have been having on you. When you reintroduce them 1 in 5, you'll find out what your system can make of them. If you react with any allergy symptoms, you need to consider taking cow's-milk dairy products out of your diet completely for as long as it takes until you no longer react severely when you test yourself with an occasional taste of cow's milk, cheese, or yogurt.

Yogurt is designated a protein, so even though it's very easy for most people to digest, I don't recommend it on cereals. It makes a good breakfast food, though, because it can be digested easily, and it can even be mixed with fruit without problems, despite the general advice that fruit should not be mixed with anything but other fruits.

Wheat also features heavily in most people's breakfasts. Wheat cereals, toast, or croissants all add to the pattern of overuse which causes many people serious health and weight-control problems. Unless it's a BFD (Best Food Day), when you are enjoying a *special* wheat breakfast, use products such as oats, whole rye bread, and crisp breads or oatcakes instead. However, try not to spread the use of these grains to other days in the week; instead keep your choice of *any* of them to the one day on which you would be using wheat. They are all grains which contain gluten, and it's best to keep gluten to one day in five.

Desserts can cause problems. Generally they're sweet, fattening, and badly combined. Most people like something sweet after a savory meal. That's not too much of a problem after carbohydrate meals, because sugar is a carbohydrate, but it can be difficult after proteins.

The best idea is to eat well from the early courses of a meal and sparingly from your dessert. That way you will enjoy it as a counterpoint or contrast to the flavors of your main courses, but won't have to rely on what are often fattening foods for a major part of your meal. If weight control is particularly important to you, try to *avoid desserts* altogether.

However, it is possible to incorporate sweet desserts into any meal by bending the rules slightly, as you will soon discover. With your Master Plan, I've taken the view that if you want the most rapid results for your health and shape, you will *avoid* sweet desserts. If you do want something sweet to finish your meal, the desserts shown are the least of all evils!

Drinks that interfere with good digestion shouldn't be used while you are eating. But some drinks can be used to assist your digestion of a meal, and some can accompany a meal without the risk they will hinder digestion.

With breakfast, choose from coffee or tea (preferably black), herb or fruit teas, and if yours is a fruit breakfast, fruit juice.

With other main meals try vegetable or tomato juice spiced with Tabasco or Worcestershire sauce if you want. These are especially good as aperitifs. Other beverages to have with a meal are wine, champagne, coffee, and tea (both preferably black).

Your Daily Menus do not show drinks because the ones mentioned here are those that would appear in every option.

Toxins released from your body by your better eating will need flushing from your system. It can be helped if you drink plenty of **water** but water hinders digestion if taken with a meal because it can dilute your stomach acid. So drink it *between* main meals so that it can help every other process in your body.

Try to drink about one and a half liters of water a day in addition to other liquids. The best way I've found of doing this is to use a one and a half liter mineral water bottle, refill it each day if you want to, and make sure you drink it all by the time you go to bed at night.

Signs that you may not be drinking enough water are strong color to your urine, a mild aching in the mid- to lower-back region, and a feeling of tightness in the abdomen, especially when you try to lie flat on your back. It will feel like your muscles are too tight to let your back be flat on the floor, and if you press your hands into your tummy, back and in toward your spine, halfway between your hip bones and the bottom edge of your ribs, it will feel tender like an aching muscle. Drinking plenty of water should resolve this.

When you have completed the fourteen days of the Master Plan, why not check up on your progress?

Check that you are maintaining your practice of affirmations and visualization. Remember, you started a thirty-day program which I am sure you will wish to finish, but notice now if your attitude or behavior is beginning to change.

Then go back to the Symptom Checklist (page 66) and give yourself new scores for today, under the Progress column. Notice what has changed and what's improved. You can return to this checklist and make a further progress check in another few weeks.

Most important of all, reinforce the new beliefs you've already introduced by *congratulating yourself* on your first fourteen days using *Love Food . . . Lose Weight*. Then make a firm decision, right now, to continue for another seven or a further fourteen days with your new way of eating.

STAYING ON TRACK

The fourteen-day Master Plan is intended as an introduction and a learning experience. To reap all the benefits of your new diet, you should continue and eventually make good food combining and food rotation your usual way of eating. This can happen almost without you realizing it on this diet.

Until you know food combining and rotation are second nature to you—and they will become so—*plan* what you intend to eat as much as possible. Use copies of the blank Five-Day Menu Arranger to make sure you have available the foods you'll need and to keep track of 1 in 5 foods. If you haven't been able to plan a meal or if you have an unplanned snack, simply record it afterward. This will help you to keep your mind focused on your chosen goals.

Only plan ahead as far as you feel comfortable. "Forever" targets have a way of disturbing your inner self—small steps can take you anywhere you want to go. There's a saying that "Success by the inch is a cinch—by the yard, it's hard." So break your big goals down into smaller, rapidly achievable ones, and just watch the progress you'll make!

The blank Daily Menu Sheet at the end of this chapter can also help you plan meals within the rules. You can create stunning new combinations to suit yourself using the ideas in the menus and recipes I've provided. You don't have to follow the daily Options exactly as they're laid out. You can choose the breakfast from either Option. You can mix and match main meals from lunch to dinner and vice versa, and between Options on the same day, without breaking the good eating rules. You can even alternate the Mix With Any starter courses and vegetable accompaniments if you prefer.

Most of the first courses, accompaniments, and even many of the desserts are Mix With Any foods that can be used with any Protein or Carbohydrate food you like. Just check to be sure they do actually combine correctly with the Protein or Carbohydrate you want to put them with.

Now let's summarize the simple rules which lie at the heart of *Love Food . . . Lose Weight*:

On Combining:

- Eat proteins and carbohydrates so they will not be present in your stomach at the same time.

On Rotation:

- All proteins, carbohydrates, and foods liable to be used on a daily basis, other than fresh fruits and Mix With Any vegetables or salads, should be eaten one day only in any five days, hence 1 in 5.

Strongly Recommended:

- Mix fruits only with other fruits, and don't mix melon with anything but other melon.

Easy, isn't it?

If you can stay within the rules about 80 percent of the time, you'll get real benefits fast. If at any time you do wander a bit too far off course, you can use this Master Plan strategy for a week or two to get back on track.

After a few months using the rules set out in these first chapters, you'll be able to relax the rules a little, and even bend them a bit. More on this later. Finally, here is the Daily Menu Sheet, which will help you to create your own meals and daily eating plans. Good luck— and *bon appétit!*

DAILY MENU SHEET FOR: _____

Breakfast	1 in 5 FOODS
Morning Snacks	
Lunch	**Stock and Shopping Checklist**
	❑
	❑
	❑
	❑
	❑
	❑
Afternoon Snacks	❑
	❑
Dinner	❑
	❑
	❑
	❑
	❑
	❑
	❑

4

Slimming the Smart Way

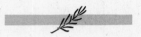

LET'S TALK ABOUT YOU

This is, of course, the chapter many people will turn to with burning interest and greatest hope. I'm not too surprised. I've lost count of how many clients I've advised over the years, but I don't recall a single one who was entirely happy about their shape or size. So I do understand the distress that can be caused by feeling your body isn't the size and shape you want it to be. It's one of the few things that can make a person consistently unhappy, or at the very least constantly frustrated. Weight and shape seem so unmanageable, yet it's important for you to be comfortable in your body and to feel in control of your appearance, isn't it?

Let's talk frankly. Like most people, you almost certainly don't understand *why* your body is its present shape. If you're not really clear about this key point, then you're probably making mistaken assumptions about what you can and should do about your figure. In fact, you've probably tried some methods to get in shape already—and met with less success than you'd like.

Most people who are anxious about their shape or size assume the problem is excess fat. They believe fat is "stuff" that sticks to their body in random lumps simply because they've eaten too much. The assumption is that fat in the body is stored energy, and since energy comes from food, all they have to do to get back to a trim, lean shape is to cut down on the calories they put in and perhaps increase the calories they burn up. A simple matter of arithmetic. Yet the equations rarely work out.

Most adults in our modern societies do have a poorer shape than they could have; they are overweight and, if you'll excuse the pun, it's a problem that's getting bigger. But the problem isn't just a matter of excess calories—that's a myth that doesn't do justice to how your body really works, and it won't give you a strategy for getting and keeping the body shape you'll be happy with.

When I massage people, my hands show me there is definitely fat under their skin, and more often than not there is more than there needs to be. But I also find excess water and fluid retention, and I find poor muscle tone and lax skin.

There are, you see, a variety of materials that produce your shape and size. There are tissues—skin, muscles, and connective membranes. There are substances held within those tissues—fat, water, and chemicals. The composition and makeup of the tissues and substances within them is highly individual. One person's muscles can be stiff and rigid, while another's are like wet spaghetti. One person may have soft tissue that allows their limbs to bend like a rubber doll, while another can barely touch their knees, let alone their toes. One person can accumulate fat around their hips while another gets fluid on their upper arms or bust.

Your body—the form those various elements have taken in the size, weight, and shape that is you—is *special*. It is the unique result of your individual physical and mental process which I've already mentioned—your personal body/mind ecology. So before you can expect to transform yourself in ways that will satisfy you, you need to understand the nature of your problem better, and learn a way to deal with it.

YOUR BODY IS APPROPRIATE

At this very moment, you are *absolutely* the right size, shape, and weight.

You may find this difficult to believe, but it's true. Before I explain the strategies to use for your weight and size, let's consider, for a moment, your body and your relationship with it. From that beginning, together we can expect to come up with a solution that will really help you become—and then remain—the shape and size you want to be.

When people say they're overweight, they usually mean that when they look in the mirror, they see parts of themselves that are bigger or floppier than they want them to be. It may be just one or two places or it may be all over, but somehow their proportions don't look right and things look out of control. People feel sensations of awkwardness, heaviness, or bloatedness about their body. They can feel distended or distorted somehow from what they feel they ought to be like regardless of whether they actually have too much fat and fluid or not.

Right now, though, your body is *absolutely* the right size, shape, and weight—it is *perfectly* suited to the physical and mental processes, the body/mind ecology, which keeps you alive. I call it the Appropriate Body Phenomenon. Your body naturally results from the process which underpins everything about you.

It's not your body's fault if it hasn't been able to produce a better shape and size. Remember how the body/mind process can spiral out of control, bringing health and weight problems in its wake? Remember how that same process prompts your eating, and when it isn't working well can produce the kind of eating we associate with excess weight? Remember how that process means every part of you influences every other part? So your thoughts and feelings are affecting the organs which distribute fats and fluids around your body, just as they are influencing the muscles which hold you erect and give you shape.

Your body right now is just as you've allowed it to become, probably because you have been unaware of how your body/mind process was affecting you. You've unknowingly sustained the inner reality of your self-image and presented it as a model for every other part and function of your personal ecology to become organized around. Your body therefore expresses, as it naturally must, the limitations of that model in your size and shape, posture and muscle tone, fat and fluid distribution.

The process which created your present body is ongoing and, if left to itself, will continue to present you with an Appropriate Body. Over the coming years that will mean an increasing girth, more fats and fluids, and reduced tone and elasticity in your muscles. However, if you *don't* have the body you want, you *can* change it—if you want to—by redirecting your inner process to provide you with a slimmer and lighter self.

That's what slimming is all about.

THE THREE CAUSES OF FATNESS

Many people think they are doomed by their genes to be fat. They believe there's little they can do about their shape, and that's why their attempts to change it don't work. Some people even lean on this idea as an excuse for doing nothing. They were "born this way," and that's all there is to it, or "My mother was overweight, so I suppose I'll end up like that too."

In fact, except for a very few people, genetic inheritance is only one factor among many that influence your size, shape, and weight. Your genes play an important role, it's true, but that role is relatively limited and one that becomes less significant as time passes.

Think, for a moment, about the huge surge in obesity in the past few years. Common sense will tell you that nothing in our genes could have changed so quickly to make humans gain so much weight over such a short period of time. Evolution simply doesn't happen that fast. Scientists can identify only a handful of genetic changes in our species, as having occurred during the last ten thousand years (that's right—ten thousand years). It's nonsense to suggest that the upsurge in obesity over the past few decades is primarily a genetic problem.

Your genes are not a blueprint with your finished dimensions set down in indelible ink. Rather, your genes lay down the guidelines by which every part of you will grow from the first cells. They establish the foundations for each part's beginnings, and the frameworks and rules within which those parts can achieve a range of possible outcomes.

How you grow and develop—from embryo to infant through childhood to adult—depends on a variety of elements. These elements, which shape and steer your personal ecology, your body/mind process, I've told you about—and you already know now that you can bring a great many of those elements *within your control.* With your Master Plan you've already begun to do so.

In yoga it's said that perfect health and fitness come from three rights—right thinking, right eating, and right exercise. Here we have a clue about how to alter and guide the process which is at the hub of your size and weight situation.

The way you characteristically think and feel about yourself, your eating, and the amount and specific ways you use your muscles are the connections between your self-image and how it manifests as your figure. You could say they are the *channels* through which your inner process produces the form you are.

Remember, you are, by nature, a living ecology: if one aspect of you is affected, all the others are affected as well. If, for instance, you improve your eating skillfully, it can help you improve your weight and shape, and also help you to improve your inner self-image. The same is true with your thinking and the way you use your body. They can all be the means to improve the way you are now, and to improve the inner process which can *keep* you as you want to be.

Addressing these three key areas together, in the right way, is what the KW slimming approach is all about and why it gives you such fantastic potential. It's a method for resolving your weight problems, and for rectifying the process behind them, in a way which will also bring benefits to your health and self-esteem.

It comes as no surprise to find that yoga, an ancient form of spiritual and physical exercise, is based on an understanding of the very deepest workings of the human system. Nor should it be surprising that the thinking, eating and the form of exercising advocated in yoga should have profound effects on health, weight, shape, and mental outlook. The yogis clearly understood human ecology and the body/mind process.

So let's look more closely at these three areas—your thinking, eating, and body use—to see what they can tell us about what's affecting your body dimensions and how to make things better for you. We'll start with your eating.

THREE WAYS TO CORRECT YOUR EATING HABITS

I've already explained quite a bit about why you eat what you do. I've shown you how your eating is intricately linked with your body/mind process, how it becomes compromised, and how it's involved in your health and weight when it goes wrong.

So let's consider your present diet. We'll make the assumption that any poor eating habit, or lopsided bias in your food intake, is both a sign and a cause of the problems which are affecting your body/mind process and of the figure-control difficulties that have arisen from it.

Check 1: Correcting Your Food Combinations

Poor food combining fulfills a necessary function badly. Poor combinations of food give your body and mind what they need but in ways your digestive system finds difficult to deal with. Over time, the effects of bad combining cause or aggravate illness and poor weight distribution.

The first and foremost solution to your weight and shape difficulties is to give yourself the foods you need *in ways your body can use easily*. There's no easier way to achieve this than with food combining, which remains a principal part of Slimming Strategies.

Check 2: Correcting Food Overuse

Some foods, if eaten too often—and daily or almost daily is too often—cause difficulties that make them a significant factor in your size, weight, and shape problems. If you take *any* food or drink, other than fresh fruit or Mix With Any vegetables and salads, in large amounts or on a frequent basis, they probably are playing a role in producing any excess weight you're carrying.

This is particularly true of grain carbohydrates, concentrated dairy foods (especially cow's dairy products), eggs, soy, beans, nuts, and a few other foods I'll cover later. Bringing these foods under control in your diet may well be the key to your problem. Overuse of some foods commonly gives rise to allergies and sensitivities which result in bloating, fluid retention, puffiness in the tissues, and loss of muscle tone. Alternatively, the food you're overusing may contain too much fat, sugar, or salt, all of which can have a direct effect on the distribution of fats or fluids on your body.

One-in-five food rotation forms a fundamental part of the basic Master Plan. It takes care of many foods which you may have been overeating, so it should remain a part of your Slimming Strategy, but there are probably other foods you are still overusing which could be the key to your weight and size improvements.

Special Slimming Strategies will help you identify the foods which could be causing you problems and help you get them under control in your diet.

Each food presents a complex story of a substance that affects both your mind and body and can directly or indirectly influence your weight and dimensions. They are substances the body can use quite well in moderation, but if eaten too often they can cause serious problems.

The list of foods which you can address in your Slimming Strategies includes some which, if taken in excess, can overstimulate systems in your body and mind or mimic the action of powerful natural substances. It doesn't take a lot of imagination to realize these effects, over time, will also be affecting your figure and your health in critical ways.

Foods you'll address on your Slimming Strategies include:

- **Caffeine**—found in coffee, tea, cola drinks, cocoa, chocolate
- **Fats and Oils**—in chocolate, cheese, and other high-fat dairy products, butter and margarine, red meats, all processed meats, junk foods and snacks such as potato or corn chips, nuts, burgers, fries, shakes, and fried foods
- **Sugar**—white or brown sugar in beverages, canned drinks, sweets, confectionery of all kinds, cakes, biscuits, cookies, dried fruits, honey, maple syrup, and molasses
- **Chocolate**—notice how it keeps cropping up!
- **Wheat**—your old enemy (see page 49), found in bread, biscuits, cakes, cookies, pasta, processed foods (I've found wheat in meat products, chocolates, and soups just as examples, so check the labels!)
- **Alcohol**—in all guises

On your slimming plan you'll identify the foods which may be causing you a problem, and you will reduce your intake of them gradually over a fixed period of time until, for a short while, you stop using them altogether.

Check 3: Correcting Food Aversion

A strong *aversion* to a food, salt for example, can indicate, as much as overuse, that something is not right in your system. You don't need to force yourself to eat anything you don't like. You may find, however, as a result of the diet or one of the Slimming Strategies that follow, you suddenly have a desire for foods you preferred not to eat before, or are developing a taste for a much wider range of foods altogether. These are signs to look for that your system is undergoing a deep and powerful transformation.

So let's move on to consider what we can learn from how you are using your muscles.

IMPROVING YOUR MUSCLES

The story of your muscles is similar in many ways to that of your eating habits. The quality and characteristics of your muscles are molded by the same organizing process that affects your eating and everything else about you—your body/mind process. The shape and quality of your muscles and how you can use them—in posture, movement, exercise—therefore become indicators of how effective the wider process is and whether problems exist within it.

You probably have some fairly clear ideas of how important to your shape and weight your muscles are, but there may be a few surprises in store for you when we look a little further.

The most obvious way in which your muscles are significant to your overall shape and size is in the contour and bulk they form over your bones. Consider, though, that while it is the amount and type of activity and exercise you regularly do which gives them their size and shape, they can't begin to reach their potential if, for some reason, they are weak, prone to injury, have poor supplies of nutrients, or can't deal well with toxins produced by exercise. In any of those circumstances you won't be able to get much shape to them at all.

Lax and weak muscles are more inclined to accommodate the presence of fats and fluids within and around them, and are less able to play an effective role in mobilizing fats and fluids when you want to shift them.

Don't forget, too, that much of this applies to facial as well as body muscle.

So what should you look for? Here are some of the muscle-related problems you might recognize.

Both tight muscles and loose muscles can result directly from the influence of your self-image. In psychology it's called "character armoring," which refers to the way muscles develop over time, in sympathy with your self-image and the thoughts and feelings you have about your self and the world around you. I call it *intrinsic body language*. It means that your attitudes toward yourself and the world are reflected in the attitude your body expresses. In other words, you acquire a pattern of tight and loose muscles that then pull your body into a *posture* characteristic of what you believe about yourself deep down inside.

The same situation is reflected in your facial muscles, which take on your habitual *expressions*. To test this out you could try pretending to be angry, then sad, then frightened and finally happy. Each time notice what happens to the muscles in your face and body. Anyone who has learned to see themselves in a way that makes them feel deeply angry, sad, frightened, or happy will eventually find their face is pulled into an appropriate expression to show those feelings.

Your self-image and its attendant emotions and thoughts also affect your organs and glands. You probably know well the effects of extreme feelings on your digestion and heart, for instance, and you've almost certainly felt the effects on your body of adrenaline and other chemicals stimulated by emotional situations.

The alternative health discipline of kinesiology teaches that each organ and gland is associated, via your energy meridian system, with certain muscles or muscle groups. Whatever affects a particular organ or gland can consequently affect its associated muscles. Persistent stomach-acid problems related to stress, for instance, could well be reflected in the muscles associated with the stomach, some of which are in your neck. Neck stiffness is indeed very common among those suffering stress-related stomach-acid problems.

Cramps are another example of muscles indicating problems else-where in your body/mind process. Probably the most common site for cramps in muscles is in those at the back of the lower leg, the calf muscles. Well-known causes of cramp are salt depletion, fluid loss, and fatigue. We can all get cramps, but particularly athletes who, in the midst of competition, feel their calf muscles become solid knots of pain, especially if they haven't drunk enough water.

Why, though, should the calf muscles be so prone to this problem? After all, don't all the leg muscles and many others get just the same amount of use? In kinesiology, your calf muscles are associated with your adrenal glands. These glands sit on top of your kidneys. They help you deal with the stress you would experience in competitive sports. Your kidneys are the organs that regulate fluid balance in your body and which become distressed by excessive fluid loss and stress. No wonder sports people get cramps in their calves.

Something else that can adversely affect your organs and glands is food. Bad eating aggravates or causes problems in your digestive organs. It can also produce toxins that can compromise various organs, or it can provoke your glands into reactions they shouldn't have to make. What-ever the result, there is every chance of a consequent reaction in the muscles related to the organs or glands affected.

Examples are *lower back pain* associated with bowel disturbances, *abdominal distension* because the small intestine is affected, and *mid-back pain* with *abdominal stiffness* caused by kidney dehydration.

If the disruption caused to the organ or gland is prolonged or per-sistent, the body reaction is likely to be *periods of localized muscular discomfort*. If the organic disruption is only sporadic, the response may be *occasional acute localized muscle pain*.

These reactions occur because individual muscles tighten or loosen in relation to other muscles around them, when their associated organ or gland is compromised. Muscles are able to hold you properly upright and move you around by being balanced in healthy tension, one with another. So *loss of tone*—that is, an inability to hold normal healthy tension—is a common consequence of many of these adverse situations. Individual muscles are effectively switched off and lose their inner strength.

Your body's natural alignment can become distorted if some mus-cles become looser or tighter than the others around them. Muscles of differing strength can work against each other, instead of with each other, to pull you out of shape into a *poor posture*.

Excessively tight muscles can give rise to persistent muscle pain anywhere in your body. The muscle is just too stiff and rigid and subject to too much stress and strain.

Excessively lax muscles can aggravate problems by exacerbating misalignment which, if it's prolonged, is likely to result in *joint pains* and even joint damage, because unevenly balanced muscles pull joints out of alignment, and moving joints when they are not properly aligned strain the surrounding soft tissues and can cause uneven wear and tear and subsequent pain.

Overly tight and overly lax muscles can be involved in *strains and sprains* from relatively light use. A muscle that's too tight is already at risk of injury, and muscles that are too loose are not playing their essential role in balancing and supporting other muscles—which are then put at risk as well.

When you exercise, or even when you move around in your everyday activity, you may well notice *excessive stiffness* and *lack of mobility* in your muscles and joints. Conversely you may realize you have the opposites—*joints which overextend* and *lack of strength*. You may be prone to *muscle or joint injuries* when you exercise, or you may find you *recover slowly* from exercise or injuries.

> A sign that your muscles are in poor condition is tenderness or soreness when they are pressed firmly (but not harshly). Healthy muscles in good condition can be pressed and squeezed firmly without causing discomfort.

All the symptoms I've mentioned are warning signs that something in your body/mind process is causing a problem with your weight control and size reduction. Each one of us is different in the precise way our muscles demonstrate that such problems exist. What I'm going to tell you now must, therefore, be tempered by what you know about your own body.

Ideally your muscles should be *pliant*—they ought to be soft and malleable but not floppy when relaxed, and elastic and firm when in use.

I remember a comment made by the wife of a famous muscular movie star. She was asked what it was like being married to the man and replied that one of her enduring delights was to wake up and "see his butt like two billiard balls lying side by side" next to her in bed. Now, I have to tell you that muscles should *not* be hard, rigid and taut, and bunched up like a sack of rocks all the time! In fact, tennis balls would be better than billiard balls—firm but squeezable.

Your muscles should make your body inviting; they should not form a barrier. You should be able to relax all your muscles when lying down comfortably, not find yourself holding some muscles tight all the time. You should not have your fingers or toes curled into claws of tension when you lie down to sleep, or feel your jaw stiff and your teeth clamped tight together. Your shoulders shouldn't be around your ears.

You are made to move. You can use movement to help you feel good. Movement tones muscles and makes fat and fluids shift around your body. Movement can massage your internal organs and stimulate your glands. Exercise can even improve your libido.

Next time you set out to walk somewhere, take the opportunity to be aware of how your muscles are working. Try exaggerating your movements a little. Feel how your calf muscles squeeze and pump to make fluids move up from your lower legs. Put your hand on your abdomen and feel the muscles working. Feel the muscles of your hips and lower back flexing and moving to form a platform from which your legs can move while keeping your upper body steady.

The better and more easily you can move, the better it is for your body shape, health, and general well-being.

Yoga is an example of how muscles and movement can exploit the body/mind process. The movement and postures of yoga massage internal organs, stimulate glands, and tone muscles. Yoga, you'll recall, is not just used for health and fitness; it's also used as a path to mental and spiritual well-being.

The Slimming Strategies show you how you can use your muscles safely and easily, for long-term weight and size control, in ways which will help your whole body/mind. You can expect to resolve many of the problems mentioned here, and improve your general health, your self-image, and outlook on life.

Before turning to that there is a third and final area in which we can look for factors associated with your size and shape.

IMPROVING YOUR MIND

Various psychologists have associated acquired weight and size to a number of mental causes. In severe instances of mental difficulty, size and weight issues can become extreme, but you don't have to suffer from chronic mental illness for your mind to play a key role in your weight and size situation. The ways you think and feel about yourself can be translated via your body/mind process into body-dimension problems of various kinds.

Becoming substantially overweight may be the outcome of behavior with food that is expressing some deeper anxiety. Use of food may, for instance, indicate manipulating or taking control of at least one element in a world that seems out of control. "I'm not in charge of what's happening to me, but at least I decide what I eat and no one can stop me doing that."

For another person who sees themselves as unlovable or threatened by close relationships, fat accumulation may be a form of self-mutilation, a way of avoiding the close attention of others. "Don't let them come too close, and they won't find out how really awful I am." Or perhaps, for someone in a relationship it's a way of testing the extent of their partner's affection. "Do you love me even when I'm like this?"

Of course, these are extreme examples, but they do illustrate that substantial aspects of inner reality and self-image exert powerful influences on the body processes. Even when the beliefs you hold about yourself are not so tyrannical, their existence is enough to cast some influence on your physique. So it's in your mind that you need to look for the real cause of any problems you may have with your weight.

I'm going to tell you what signals your mind can give you. To be more accurate, I'll show what to look for in the thoughts, feelings, ideas, beliefs, attitudes, and assumptions that emanate from your inner self.

I cannot make the connections for you, however. That would

require a knowledge of you personally and a degree of analysis which are not appropriate here. Your mind gives specific signals which only you can correlate to your personal behavior or to a particular outcome in your body. You must be your own observer and evaluate what you find.

Here's what to look for.

We speak to ourselves in our minds all the time. Sometimes you have a dialogue with yourself; sometimes you rehearse what you're going to say or write down. Sometimes you give yourself commands, edicts, criticism, encouragement—in fact, all that goes to make up verbal human communication also goes on in your head.

You chat, discuss, babble, argue, joke, swear, and recite in voices that are children, parents, adults, teachers, wise people, and fools. It's called inner dialogue, and it's another manifestation of all the many facets of your inner self.

By stepping back from your inner dialogue, and being objective about what you hear, you'll find out what attitudes, assumptions, and beliefs are most frequently behind your actions and behavior. We all tend to promote certain traits of our self-image over others. The traits that seem to be most useful dominate and become the most influential; their voices in our inner dialogue are the loudest.

For example, at some time you may have accepted the belief that you should put others before yourself, maybe as a means of getting their admiration and approval. Your inner dialogue will reflect that and may even be in the tone of voice of the person from whom, years ago, you learned such an idea.

Your inner dialogue will repeat this message using language, figures of speech, and phrases that belittle yourself and insist you act in ways that are self-deprecating. Let's take this example a little further, because it's a common situation. A belief that you are less important than others—your partner, your children, your parents, your friends—usually means you put them higher than yourself on your unconscious list of priorities. You then wake up one morning and find yourself supporting this great crowd of people and wondering why your self-neglect has left you exhausted, fat, and resentful. You can't quite put your finger on what you're angry at because the world is just the way it ought to be, you're doing just what you ought to be doing, and you ought to be grateful . . . shouldn't you?

By noticing what and how you are communicating to yourself in your inner dialogue, you'll be able to ask: "Is this really the way it ought to be, or is there a better way that will lead to a better figure and maybe a happier and more healthy life?"

In your inner dialogue, then, you may become aware of language which is persistently *negative*, and words that constantly *diminish you* in any way. Listen for statements that *undervalue* you or command you to be or act *subordinate* when it's not appropriate. Listen for the *ought to* and *should be* that are the language of imposed authority from long ago, not the voices of your own self-caring reason. "Eat it all up or you'll never be big and strong," or "If you don't like what I've cooked for you, then you don't really love me," or "Children should do what they're told and not what they want—eat your bread."

Hear the dialogue that insists *you aren't good enough* or *other people are better* than you. Notice if you hear yourself constantly saying you *don't deserve* or *could have done better*.

Your inner dialogue may be in the tone or language of authoritarian parents or teachers or be like that of a child. These are characteristic of the source of the belief they express. Sources from your past which have remained unquestioned until now, and are certainly out of date.

Become aware, too, of the feelings that go with the dialogue. Your inner dialogue will be accompanied by emotions because that's where emotions originate. They are intrinsic parts of your self-image.

You may be saying to yourself, once again, that you *shouldn't make a fuss*, while you're feeling an all too familiar intense rage at being ignored, or fobbed off—as usual, Goddammit!

Notice what you are feeling, whether it's congruent with what your inner dialogue is saying, and if the intensity of the emotion is appropriate to the thought or situation which generated it. Sense whether the emotion is one you rarely experience or if you're accustomed to it. You may have accepted fear, anxiety, resentment, or sadness as the normal background to your inner discussion.

Your inner self-model will also express itself in the language you speak out loud to others. You can review it and assess for yourself whether it's supportive of you or not, in the same way as you can with your inner dialogue. It may well indicate beliefs and attitudes that, unknown to you, are factors in your weight problems.

You could be surprised at the words you most often use in normal conversation. They can indicate problems with your self-esteem and self-image, or show a deep lack of self-respect.

For instance, notice *self-denigrating* language that always puts others' interests before your own. Hear yourself use inappropriate words that are out of context, such as hate or anger. If you say, "I'm dying for an ice cream" or "I hate people who have nose hair" or "I could kill him for saying he doesn't like my hair," do you mean it?

It may sound insignificant, but do it all the time, and the message you're giving to your self-image, your inner self, is only too clear.

Try to be aware if you're *suppressing* or *denying* your real emotions when you speak to others. So often we can say one thing and feel another. Outside: "Oh, yes, that's fine, go right ahead." Inside: "Aaargh, why me?"

Your self-image is your framework of experience and your reference for new choices. You turn to it when you have to make a decision. It communicates by your inner dialogue and your feelings. Your thoughts offer the reasoning about what you should and shouldn't do.

It's the way you choose what actions to take and not to take, and it's the basis for your habitual behavior. If you have a belief system that says, "I will always fail," then you will probably not try new things or fail if you do.

You can notice in your behavior and choices the influence of your inner self-image. Notice when you *always put other people's interests before your own*, or if you *always avoid new experiences*. Do you usually dismiss the possibility that you can succeed?

Lethargy and lard go hand in hand! If you want to know why you may have acquired the attributes of a couch potato, you can find the answers in the inner dialogue you hear when you're thinking why you should and why you needn't bother exercising. You might find your answers in the words you use when you're telling someone else why you aren't going to go swimming. You might be *motivated to fail* by your own inner self.

Your mind is where your excess weight has its origins. The seeds of your failure to control your size are rooted there. And that's where you need to plant the *seeds of your success* if you are to become slimmer and stay slimmer.

There is one "right thinking" issue that does need bringing to your attention. I know that the shape and size one person can be really unhappy about is just the kind of body another would give their eye teeth for. That raises several very interesting questions. Are you really fat, or do you just think you are? Is your body really as bad as you believe it is, or is your dissatisfaction with it a sign of a more general dissatisfaction with your life and outlook?

The keys to achieving the body you'll like involve more than just knowing how to change what you are—they include *knowing how to like the shape and size you are capable of achieving*.

I'm not trying to convince you that you don't have a size or weight problem to take care of—most of us do. I am putting into context a problem that most people see far too simplistically, and in doing so never find a solution with which they'll be content.

Either they have a good image of what their body can be but fail to find the strategy that will produce and maintain it; or they have a problem accepting the best they can achieve and so cannot be happy no matter what they look like. Part of the solution to your dissatisfaction with your body is knowing yourself better and making decisions about changing yourself from a viewpoint (a self-image) of self-acceptance and knowledgeable self-care.

Despite its crucial importance, your mind is the most neglected aspect of most diets and weight-control programs. But not with *Love Food . . . Lose Weight*. With the Slimming Strategies you'll be working *with* your mind to make your body slimmer.

WEIGHT CONTROL THE LOVE FOOD . . . LOSE WEIGHT WAY

Now I want to show you precisely how you can use *Love Food . . . Lose Weight* to take permanent control of your weight, size, and shape.

The initial Master Plan you've already taken on board is a basic use of methods designed to put an end to the most common eating mistakes which are so often the cause of weight and size problems. It also improves the underlying body/mind process from which those difficulties arise, so—slowly and surely—your weight and size problems are *already* being sorted out. The conditions for a more appropriate weight and shape are gradually being established all the time you are eating well the *Love Food . . . Lose Weight* way.

But this book can take you *further still* toward your goal for a better body. Its fundamental approach can be modified to even greater effect—either to hurry things along, or to conquer a particularly tenacious weight/size situation. Let me show you now how to fine-tune this diet to transform even more rapidly and powerfully your unique shape problem.

As you now know, three main areas have to be reorganized to support your best shape and size—eating, muscles, and mind. You've already gone a long way with your eating and mind, but you can do even better. At the same time, you'll discover how to add the final element essential to a better body—exercise—until you have the most effective plan you can use for dealing with your unique body shape problem.

INTRODUCING STRATEGIES

Here are three Strategies—short, thirty-day plans for systematically changing the circumstances that keep you overweight or out of shape. Each strategy enables you to do three very important things at the same time:

- First, you'll rapidly improve your size and shape by using exercises and eating patterns that will work directly on the actual body situation you're experiencing.
- Second, with exercises and mind-management techniques that act deeply throughout your system, you'll improve the body/mind process that underpins your current situation.
- Third, your Strategy—and all of your previous *Love Food . . . Lose Weight* experience—will add new and important information to the growing resource of knowledge you hold about your body and mind. In years to come, despite new circumstances and the effects of time on your body, you'll have a *deep understanding* of how to maintain your size and shape.

Each Strategy is a complete program, targeting a particular type of figure problem. All the Strategies address the three main elements involved in size or shape difficulties: your eating, your muscles, and your mind-set. Combining effective techniques for all these elements, and aiming them specifically at the one issue that is your main problem, gives you an immensely powerful tool for bringing the situation under control once and for all.

I'm going to show you how to choose precisely which Strategy is the most appropriate to give yourself that decisive push toward a better body. From it, your quest for a slimmer, more active form will accelerate rapidly toward your goal. Even when you resume regular *Love Food . . . Lose Weight* eating, the ripples of your Strategy will act throughout your system long after your Strategy's brief duration.

The three Strategies deal with excess fat, excess fluid, and poor muscle quality. You probably already have a good idea which is most relevant to you. The questionnaire that follows will enable you to identify even more clearly which of the three Strategies you need to use first.

Of course, it's possible that more than one of these problems is contributing simultaneously to your excess weight or poor shape. The best thing you can do is to identify your *main* problem and deal with that first. If any other problem remains, you can use another strategy later and reap even more benefits.

Here's the questionnaire—put a tick in the box alongside the statements which seem most relevant to you.

THE STRATEGY CHOOSER

Statement	Check here if appropriate	
I believe my main problem is excess fat (in my diet or on my body).		A
I often feel very thirsty, or I feel very uncomfortable drinking water.		B
I have little energy and am not inclined to be active.		C
I often eat high-fat foods particularly with carbohydrates (i.e., desserts).		A
I often eat starchy meals (i.e., baked potato).		B

THE STRATEGY CHOOSER

Statement	Check here if appropriate	
I believe my main problem is poor muscle quality.		C
I often find myself feeling angry or aggressive for no reason.		A
I eat a lot of salty foods or, conversely, cannot eat anything salty.		B
I often suffer from aching muscles.		C
I often suffer from indigestion.		A
I believe my main problem is excess fluid.		B
I have poor posture and do not feel comfortable standing for a long time.		C
I do not like fatty foods and may even feel nauseated by the thought of them.		A
I often feel emotionally sensitive for little reason, or conversely I have few emotional reactions.		B
I usually lack confidence and have low self-esteem.		C

Count how many checks you've put for questions marked A, B, and C respectively and enter your scores in the boxes below.

	A	B	C
YOUR SCORE			

If you checked more A statements than any other, you should follow the Fat Burner Strategy.

Excess fat under the skin differs in quality and consistency from person to person and even from place to place on the same person. Generally, though, the amount of excess is fairly consistent once it's established.

Fat is less dense than muscle but more dense than fluid and usually adheres quite closely to the skin that covers it. Fat can cause the skin to have a variety of surfaces that resemble pitting, denting, or the well-known orange peel effect, each of which can vary from slight to extreme and seem worse when the skin is grasped and bunched up.

If you've scored more B's, you need the Fluid Reduction Strategy.

If you have too much fluid, you'll find it much easier to lift your skin away from the underlying muscles and there will be a definite sense of fluid between skin and underlying muscles. If you tap yourself in some places, you may even see ripples travel under your skin in much the same way as when you disturb any collection of water.

Fluid retention fluctuates. There is usually a level of excess that's fairly constant, but after meals, at the end of the day, or after a long journey, for instance, you're likely to find even more has accumulated and you'll weigh two or three pounds more than in the morning. You may also find the excess water gathers in particular places. Fluid is affected more by gravity than is fat or muscle, so your body can "slip south" slightly during the day if excess fluid is your main problem.

Obviously, quite a lot of the fluid on your body is transitory. You'll notice that you have "good body" days and "bad body" days. Your "best body" is usually the one you find first thing in the morning, after a night's sleep during which your sensitive fluid balance has remained undisturbed by any of the elements that can stir it up.

If you've checked mostly C statements, your plan is to follow the Muscle Reshaping Strategy.

Muscle quality also differs considerably from person to person, and assessing your own muscles by touch is difficult. It's rather like trying to tickle yourself: your muscles simply don't cooperate. They cannot be active *and* completely relaxed at the same time.

You can determine more about your muscle quality by how comfortable they feel, how you look in your normal postures, and how they respond to use. If, when standing, your stomach sticks out a lot, especially after meals, then your muscles may have lost integrity, perhaps because of what you've eaten. If your abdomen sticks out constantly and at the same time your lower back is curved inward, it's likely you have weak muscles in either or both areas. Consistently poor posture is a strong sign of poor muscle quality.

Similarly, if you react badly to even gentle exercise—rapidly experiencing burning or aching, or perhaps incurring strains and sprains very easily—then your muscles are probably weaker than they ought to be. Key signs of poor muscle quality are:

- If you take more than forty-eight hours to recover from even light exercise.
- If you suffer aching in your lower back, hips, or legs after standing still for a while.
- If your muscle definition is poor. You won't be able to distinguish by observation or touch individual muscles in a group like those in your thigh; instead they'll seem like a single ill-defined mass.

If you found the questionnaire was inconclusive, choose the Strategy you feel to be most relevant. Each Strategy deals to some extent with all the problems; their benefits overlap.

So, write down the Strategy you'll be using and the main problem you'll be dealing with:

My weight-control Strategy is . . . . . for dealing with my . . . .

Each Strategy is a complete, easy-to-follow program with full instructions and you'll soon be starting yours, but as with the Master Plan, it's important to undertake some preparations first.

ADVICE FROM YOUR DIET COACH

No self-respecting team goes into a game without a preparatory talk from their coach. If you want to *win* this game, there's little point in hurtling into your special Strategy without also taking a moment to do some basic planning. You know the value of good preparation from your practice of the *Love Food . . . Lose Weight* diet, and you also know that a systematic approach will keep you on track if your enthusiasm ebbs at any time.

Start by picking a convenient date on which to begin your Strategy. You can then prepare for your program and get used to the idea of becoming slimmer. Write your starting date here:

> **The starting date for my Slimming Strategy is . . . .**

Your chosen Strategy will last for thirty days, and will be divided into three periods of ten days. Each ten-day period will enable you to increase the effectiveness of your program by gradual increments. If you do not feel ready or comfortable about increasing your commitment after any ten-day period, you can simply repeat the ten days you've just completed instead. You'll still benefit even if you just do the first ten-day period three times over.

You must be the arbiter of your own procedure. No one else can tell you what your health, your age, and your fitness level will enable you to do. Your Strategy is designed to be safe, effective, and simple, but you should work with your weight and shape at a level with which you are comfortable.

Your Strategy has instructions and advice about special eating tactics, exercises, and mind processes. A day-to-day progress chart will enable you to keep to your program quite easily.

Your eating over the thirty days of your Strategy includes the basic food combining and food rotation you already know so well. In addition, you'll be given a list of special foods that, over the thirty days, you'll progressively reduce until, in the final ten-day period, you'll delete them entirely from your diet. You'll have full directions about what to do, and at any time in the future you'll be able to use the same method to challenge your use of any food you may think is a problem for you. Cow's milk, for example. You'll also be given suggestions for some helpful foods to *emphasize* in your diet during these thirty days. Remember, though, because your aim is to become slimmer, you should avoid overeating, focus on the new eating patterns, and whenever possible eat a little less than you have been.

The exercises you'll be using are simple and straightforward and are described in detail for you. You may think they seem too simple and are therefore unlikely to be effective. Don't be fooled! They are chosen for the powerful way they can tap into the deepest aspects of your body/mind process.

If you haven't exercised much in recent years, you will almost certainly find a little aching and tightening after your first session or two, even though the exercises may seem quite innocuous. If you follow the program accurately, any reaction is not likely to last much more than twenty-four hours. Your muscles will soon respond and adapt: you may feel the burn, but you won't catch fire!

There's a considerable difference between the natural reaction of your muscles to an unusual new level of activity and the pains from injuries or other more serious problems in muscles or joints. Be sensible. Unless you are qualified to do so, don't increase the program even though it may not seem as if you are working hard—believe me, you will be doing enough to get the response you need. Don't take chances. If you feel pain that clearly isn't just muscle fatigue, don't continue until you are satisfied it is sensible for you to do so. If you're worried you may have a serious problem, consult a health specialist before proceeding.

If you are fit and used to exercise, you may want to add more activity into your program. You'll find places where you can write in extra exercises; if you do so, set reasonable targets. Start at a level you are used to and increase in moderate increments in subsequent ten-day periods.

Finally, to do with muscles: stand your stuff and walk your talk! Remember the New You you aim to create. It's no good aspiring to a new shape and improved figure if you're still going to slop and slouch around with the same "woe-is-me" body language you may always have used. Stand as tall as you comfortably can, straighten your shoulders, breathe in deep, and lift your head up so your line of vision is outward. Be curious about what's around you. See and be seen!

Your posture is an important tool in helping your muscles and your self-image take on new qualities. You'll feel so much better if you let your body talk the language you want to hear yourself and your mind speak.

Your mind is important to anything you want to achieve, including success at your Weight Control Strategy. To establish what you want in your inner self-image, I've created a new affirmation for each Strategy, which you may use as it stands or as a basis for a more personal one you devise for yourself. Use your affirmation in the same way as you've learned already. Write it down ten times each night, and say it out loud regularly for the thirty days of your Strategy. Write it on a colored card and carry it with you. Post pieces of the same colored card where you will see them regularly. You know how (see page 62)!

Your affirmation is one way of communicating with your self-image so it will reorganize your body/mind to produce the outcome you want. Another way of making that communication is to use a visualization procedure like the one you used in your Master Plan (page 63). Here's a variation specially for your Strategy.

Remember, your inner organization must be directed toward your intended goal, the hoped-for end result. Visualization provides a clear image of what you intend and what you expect your body/mind process to achieve. Here's what to do.

Just before you start your Strategy, preferably the night before, find a quiet place where you won't be interrupted for ten minutes or so. Settle into a comfortable chair—one that's quite upright and has arm rests is ideal—or stretch out flat on the floor with a small cushion under your head. Then close your eyes, breathe deeply in and out, ten times, and imagine yourself standing in a favorite place—a beach, a cliff top, a dance floor, a playing field—anywhere that holds a strong, positive significance for you. Now begin to silently recite your affirmation. And as you recite it, imagine that your affirmation gradually begins to come true and that your body changes accordingly. Imagine that what you "see" is actually a film, one you are both directing and playing the lead role in. As the director, you are controlling through your affirmation; as the actor, you are becoming all that the affirmation promises until, at the end of the film, you have created in your mind's eye a vision of yourself as you want to be.

Now run your film again. Start at the beginning—you as you are, in a favorite place. Then see yourself gradually changing as your affirmation takes effect and slowly transforms you. Finally, see yourself as you want to be. Finish with a bold, happy moment—smile a broad happy smile of success—and cut! That's your film—that's your slimming visualization.

When you create this visualization, "see" a vision of your new self as clearly as you can and allow yourself to believe you can be that way. Don't try to work out precisely how or when you might achieve your goal but concentrate on details. "See" your shape as you imagine it could be, "see" yourself standing and moving as you would stand and move if you were the way you'd like to be. Imagine how it would feel if your body was that way. Sense what thoughts and feelings the you of your image has, and experience in your own mind the self-esteem and self-image your visualized self would enjoy.

Use this "film" as often as you like over the next thirty days. Whenever you need to reassure yourself of your intentions, run the film, and smile the smile! Whenever you are exercising or preparing food, run the film—smile the smile! Whenever you have a moment in which to recite your affirmation, run the film—smile! Whenever you find yourself in need of a little lift, run the film . . . and smile the smile of success!

The more "real" you can make the images within your film, and the more clearly you can "see" yourself, the stronger will be the directive you'll be giving to the unconscious process, from which your body shape arises.

Above all, aim for an image you can achieve. You can always reassess and repeat this procedure with new and gradually upgraded images after each small step toward your goal is completed. In filming terms, you can always do an edit! Several short and certain steps toward your goal are more effective than attempting a huge, hopeful leap. The means and the time it takes to achieve what you want must be left to the innate intelligence and natural process of your body and mind. Your Strategy, though, is the first step and a potent demonstration of your intent to become what you have envisaged within your film.

When you've completed your visualization, your filmmaking, tick the appropriate box in the Mind over Matter section of the instructions and guidelines of your Strategy. You're now ready to start creating the body you want!

Smile—you're on your way!

THE FAT BURNER STRATEGY

The aim of this thirty-day Strategy is to kick-start your body's own mechanisms which deal with fats in your system. Your body has already adopted a poor use of fats and will quickly adapt to any new methodical use of fats and oils in order to maintain its fat store. You need to profoundly *alter* these patterns in order to stimulate a more efficient fat metabolism.

Your thirty-day Fat Burner Strategy is shown below, in the form of a detailed schedule on which you will record your daily progress. It's simplicity itself to follow, but first you should read the guidelines, explanations of terms used, and instructions which follow.

Eating for Fat Burning

Use the Five-Day Menu Arranger which follows to make a five-day eating plan you can repeat throughout the thirty days following the Vital Planning Points which follow. You can do this easily by choosing low-fat options from your Master Plan menus, and adapting your cooking methods and dressings as suggested below. For example, make soups into protein, low-fat soups by replacing cream with skim or semi-skim milk, and by steaming or broiling where the recipe suggests frying.

As you can see from your daily schedule, there are occasional High-calorie days when all the usual restrictions seem to go out the window, followed by Low-calorie days when it's suggested you radically cut down on your energy intake from food.

Emphatic calorie shifts like these are used to provoke your metabolism into extra activity, and to stop it settling too comfortably into a new routine. Your body can quickly adjust to any consistently lower intake of calories and then continue to "store some away for you." Just what you *don't* want!

On High-calorie days you can eat fried foods, red meats, cheeses, oil-based dressings on salads—as long as you do so within correct food-combining and rotating principles, but you *must* continue to *avoid* fat with carbohydrate combinations at all times.

On Low-calorie days, eat lightly from calorie-scarce meals such as high-water-content fresh fruit, salads, vegetables, soups, and vegetable juices. I suggest you use the Daily Menu Planner to plan one Low-calorie day which you can turn to on the relevant days in your thirty-day Strategy.

Below you'll find some special advice which will help you with this and in planning your day's food intake for the thirty days of your Fat Burner Strategy.

THE FAT BURNER FIVE-DAY MENU ARRANGER

	KW	DAY 1	DAY 2	DAY 3	DAY 4	DAY 5
Breakfast						
Snacks						
Lunch						
Snacks						
Dinner						
Snacks						
Summary 1 in 5 Foods Used						

Options for your first day might look like this:

FAT BURNER DAILY MENU—DAY 1

	Option A	Option B
Breakfast	Fresh fruits (F) Your choice of at least three different varieties Choose drinks from fresh fruit or vegetable juice, herb or fruit teas	Mixed stewed fruit with oat bran (F)
Morning Snacks	Choose snacks from fresh fruits or crudités and drinks from the list given for breakfast	
Lunch	Mushroom soup (M/A) soups to be made with skim milk Millet or buckwheat (C) and steamed vegetables with fresh tomato and herb sauce Green salad with lemon juice and cinnamon (M/A)	Spinach and pea soup (M/A) Steamed salmon (P) and vegetable with watercress sauce (substitute milk for cream) Raw shredded veg with chopped tomato and basil dressing (M/A)
Afternoon Snacks	Choose snacks from fresh fruits or crudités and drinks from the list given for breakfast	
Dinner	Poached trout on mixed green leaves (P) Grilled turkey on ribbon vegetables with lemon juice and fresh herbs (P) Coleslaw and spinach salad with lemon juice and nutmeg (M/A)	Leek and parsnip soup (substitute milk for cream) (M/A) Whole rye bread with roasted mixed sweet peppers and tomatoes (C) Tomato and sweet onion salad with tomato juice and basil dressing (M/A)
Your 1 in 5 foods	Non-gluten grain: Millet or buckwheat Trout Turkey	Gluten grain: oat bran or rye Salmon

Fat Burner Strategy—Vital Planning Points

- **Always!** Follow strict food-combining rules (see page 43) and basic 1 in 5 food rotation
- **Never!** Combine fats or oils with carbohydrate/starchy foods. Especially avoid high-fat foods with carbohydrates.
- **Use!** Low-fat cooking such as steaming, broiling, and boiling. Emphasize these foods: fruit and/or stewed fruit breakfasts with flaxseed or oat bran; oats, brown rice, fresh fruit, vegetables and salads including raw vegetables, low-fat proteins such as low-oil fish, chicken, and turkey. Use vegetable juices, lemon juice, and fresh herbs for dressing salads. Maintain high fluid intake—drink at least two liters of fluids per day.
- **Reduce!** Fats and oils, wheat, caffeine in your daily schedule.

  Reduce by half means you should aim to reduce your average daily intake in the first ten days to approximately half your previous daily average intake of the specified food. In the second ten days you should aim for a further reduction, again halving your daily intake so that it is approximately one-quarter your initial intake. The goal is to gradually reduce your intake until, in the final ten days, you delete the specified food(s) as completely as possible from your diet.

  Suggestions: replace high-fat foods such as red meat, processed meats, cheeses, dairy products, fat spreads, chocolate, avocados, nuts, and oily fish—with different low-fat foods or low-fat options of the same item. Gradually reduce the number of days on which you use wheat and caffeine. Use non-wheat substitutes such as oat crackers or rye bread and crackers for wheat products and corn or buckwheat pasta for wheat pasta. Substitute non-caffeine and decaffeinated products, juices, herbs, and coffee substitutes for caffeine drinks.

Using Your Muscles for Fat Burning

- **Speed Walking** Find a suitable route on which to take your speed walks. Start off slowly and gradually increase speed so you warm up during the first third or quarter of your walk. In the middle part of your walk, about half the time given, walk as fast as you can while keeping good form and style. Keep your body erect, your chin up, and eyes looking straight ahead; keep your arms partially bent but swinging well like a relaxed march. Slow down in the final third or quarter of your speed walk period so you cool down gradually. Walk without any motive other than to exercise—don't use your speed walk for going somewhere or for shopping. Walk purposefully. Repeat your affirmation to the cadence of your walking. Run the film! Smile your "success" smile! Special note: be sure to wear good-purpose shoes such as trainers for your exercises.

- **Virtual Skipping** This is skipping or jumping rope without the rope. Just let your imagination take over and think about what children and boxers do with a skipping rope—except you can't get it tangled in your feet. Remember to use your arms and wrists to twirl the imaginary rope and jump or skip on the spot, on one or both feet, using any and all the fancy combinations or elaborations you can imagine. Have fun— follow the Safety Tip below.

- **Special Exercises** This heading includes a variety of exercises to stimulate your body/mind process. Take as long as you need to complete the time or number of repetitions required by your schedule without overtiring or losing good form. Yours are:

❑ *Abdominal Contraction* Lie flat on your back on a soft mat or folded towel to protect the base of your spine. Bend your legs and put the soles of your feet flat on the ground, about shoulder-width apart. This is your start position. The action is to contract your abdominal muscles as if to lift your shoulders. It's very important you do two things to minimize any strain to your neck and back. First, tip your head back a little and focus on a spot behind you throughout the exercise. Second, keep your back flat on the floor as if the back of your navel were pressing onto your spine. The action will be enough to contract your muscles without you having to lift your body at all. Hold the contracted position for three seconds before relaxing completely back to the start position. Repeat as many times as your schedule requires.

❑ *Pull Overs* Lie flat on your back, knees bent, feet flat and shoulder-width apart as you did for the Abdominal Contractions. Place a cushion on your thighs. Grasp the cushion between the palms of your hands so your arms are now stretched out. This is your start position. The action is to slowly raise your still straight arms until they are stretched up alongside your ears and the cushion is over the top of your head, a nearly semicircular movement. Hold for three seconds and slowly bring your arms back to the start position, keeping your arms straight and the cushion between your palms; rest. Repeat as many times as your schedule requires.

❑ *Cobra* Kneel on your mat with your legs together and the tops of your feet flat beneath you. Sit back on your heels and bend forward until your chest is on your thighs. Put your forearms, slightly apart, flat on the floor out in front of you in a prayer-like position and relax completely. This is your start position. The action is to slowly raise your body and hinge forward so your weight is on your hands and knees. Adjust your hands if you need to, so you have your weight comfortably in control. Keep moving forward until you can straighten your arms and drop your pelvis forward to the floor; this will cause your back to arch inward. Your weight will now be on your hands and the whole of your upper legs. Your body will be in a head-up, chest-forward, legs-flat-on-the-floor position like a cobra. Hold for three seconds and then return slowly to your start position. Relax completely. Practice once to settle in your mind what to do, then repeat as many times as your schedule requires.

• **Your Choice Exercises** There is a space in your Strategy for you to write in and record your own exercise preferences, should you already exercise regularly. If you do, you might want to try something different. Your body soon adapts to what it is used to, and fails to get the same benefits from your usual exercises. Try speed swimming (but make sure you swim properly, which means getting your head in the water), jogging, and aerobics. However, please note that heavy exercise such as aerobics or weight training is more useful for fluid reduction than fat reduction.

- **Rest Days** These are days in your schedule when you do not exercise so your body can assimilate what you've done and can deal with accumulated toxins in your muscles.

Safety Tip: To test that you are working to the right level, make certain that you can talk or sing with just a *hint* of breathlessness while you exercise. Exerting yourself to that point and no further is an easy-to-measure guide to keep you within safe limits. If you cannot talk or sing while you exercise, stop or slow down!

Your Mind over Your Matter

- **Visualization** Check here when you've completed your visualization exercise and have a full-color, action-packed film you can run whenever you like. ❏
- **Affirmation** Check here when you have created your own affirmation or have learned the affirmation provided for this Strategy and written it on each ten-day schedule in the box provided. ❏

My suggestion: "Every day little by little I RELEASE the excess FAT from my body."

(See earlier guidelines on using your affirmation to best effect.)

Follow your daily Fat Burning Schedules by looking at the instructions in the column for each day and give yourself a check when you've completed them. For example "Reduce Fats/Oils by Half"—when you've done it, give yourself a check, and so on until you've completed the last day. If you have any questions, refer back to the guidelines and instructions.

FAT BURNER DAYS 1–10

	1	2	3	4	5	6	7	8	9	10
Eating										
Reduce fats/oils by half	□	□	□	■	□	□	□	□	■	□
Reduce wheat by half	□	□	□	■	□	□	□	□	■	□
Reduce caffeine by half	□	□	□	■	□	□	□	□	■	□
High-calorie day	■	■	■	□	■	■	■	■	□	■
Low-calorie day	■	■	■	■	□	■	■	■	■	□
Exercise										
Speed walking (5 minutes)	□	□	□	■	□	□	□	□	■	□
Virtual skipping (3 minutes)	□	□	□	■	□	□	□	□	■	□
Abdominal contractions (10 times)	□	□	□	■	□	□	□	□	■	□
Pull overs (10 times)	□	□	□	■	□	□	□	□	■	□
Cobra (5 times)	□	□	□	■	□	□	□	□	■	□
Choice of exercises	□	□	□	■	□	□	□	□	■	□
Rest day	■	■	■	□	■	■	■	□	■	■
Mind over Matter										
Write your affirmation here:										
Affirmation (write/say 10 times)	□	□	□	□	□	□	□	□	□	□

Check each box when you've completed the assignment to which it refers.

FAT BURNER DAYS 11–20

	11	12	13	14	15	16	17	18	19	20
Eating										
Reduce fats/oils by half again	❑	❑	❑	■	❑	❑	❑	❑	■	❑
Reduce wheat by half again	❑	❑	❑	■	❑	❑	❑	❑	■	❑
Reduce caffeine by half again	❑	❑	❑	■	❑	❑	❑	❑	■	❑
High-calorie day	■	■	■	❑	■	■	■	■	❑	■
Low-calorie day	■	■	■	■	❑	■	■	■	■	❑
Exercise										
Speed walking (7 minutes)	❑	❑	❑	❑	■	❑	❑	❑	❑	❑
Virtual skipping (5 minutes)	❑	❑	❑	❑	■	❑	❑	❑	❑	❑
Abdominal contractions (15 times)	❑	❑	❑	❑	■	❑	❑	❑	❑	❑
Pull overs (10 times)	❑	❑	❑	❑	■	❑	❑	❑	❑	❑
Cobra (7 times)	❑	❑	❑	❑	■	❑	❑	❑	❑	❑
Choice of exercises	❑	❑	❑	❑	■	❑	❑	❑	❑	❑
Rest day	■	■	■	■	❑	■	■	■	■	■
Mind over Matter										
Write your affirmation here:										
Affirmation (write/ say 10 times)	❑	❑	❑	❑	❑	❑	❑	❑	❑	❑

Check each box when you've completed the assignment to which it refers.

FAT BURNER DAYS 21–30

	21	22	23	24	25	26	27	28	29	30
Eating										
Delete as much fat/oils as you can	❑	❑	❑	❑	❑	❑	❑	❑	❑	❑
Delete as much wheat as you can	❑	❑	❑	❑	❑	❑	❑	❑	❑	❑
Delete as much caffeine as you can	❑	❑	❑	❑	❑	❑	❑	❑	❑	❑
Exercise										
Speed walking (10 minutes)	■	❑	❑	❑	■	❑	❑	❑	❑	❑
Virtual skipping (7 minutes)	■	❑	❑	❑	■	❑	❑	❑	❑	❑
Abdominal contractions (20 times)	■	❑	❑	❑	■	❑	❑	❑	❑	❑
Pull overs (20 times)	■	❑	❑	❑	■	❑	❑	❑	❑	❑
Cobra (10 times)	■	❑	❑	❑	■	❑	❑	❑	❑	❑
Choice of exercises	■	❑	❑	❑	■	❑	❑	❑	❑	❑
Rest day	❑	■	■	■	❑	■	■	■	■	■
Mind over Matter										
Write your affirmation here:										
Affirmation (write/ say 10 times)	❑	❑	❑	❑	❑	❑	❑	❑	❑	❑

Check each box when you've completed the assignment to which it refers.

Weight and Size Progress Chart

Weigh and measure yourself first thing on the mornings shown, before any food or drink. Make sure you measure in the same place at each location on your body.

Day	1	4	7	11	14	17	21	25	28	30
Weight										
Neck										
Bust/Chest										
Waist										
Hips										
Buttocks										

THE FLUID REDUCTION STRATEGY

Your body has already adopted a poor use of water and will quickly adapt to any new methodical pattern of fluid use in order to maintain its stored fluids. You need to *alter* these patterns and stimulate the mechanisms which reduce fluids in your system. Your schedule will show occasional High-water days on which, in addition to your normal daily fluid intake, you will be asked to flush your system by drinking at least one and a half liters of water during a single half hour period. These days will be followed by Low-water days during which you will reduce your fluid intake to half a liter.

Just like the Fat Burner Strategy, your Fluid Reduction Strategy is in the form of a detailed schedule on which you will record your daily progress. Here are the instructions, guidelines, and explanations of the terms used in your Fluid Reduction Strategy.

Fluid Retention Strategy—Vital Planning Points

- Use the Five-Day Menu Arranger (page 90) to plan your eating for each day, making sure you follow the strategy outlined for the day on the Fluid Reduction schedule below.

- **Always!** Follow strict food-combining rules (see page 36) and basic 1 in 5 food rotation. Maintain a high fluid intake—drink plenty of fluids each day and at least one and a half liters of plain water, except on High- or Low-water days indicated in your daily schedule.
- **Use!** Moist cooking methods such as steaming, boiling, microwave, and stir-fry. A high-protein diet with plenty of salads and vegetables to help you cut down intake of all types of carbohydrates. Fresh fruit, vegetables, and salads including raw vegetables. Flaxseeds or oat bran with fresh or stewed fruits for breakfasts. Fluid-reducing foods such as basil, parsley, beetroot, fennel, and celery seeds in cooking.
- **Reduce!** Salt, wheat, caffeine, alcohol in your daily schedule.

  Reduce by half means you should aim to reduce your average daily intake in the first ten days to approximately half your previous daily average intake of the specified food. In the second ten days you should aim for a further reduction again, halving your daily intake so that it is approximately one-quarter your initial intake. The goal is to gradually reduce your intake until, in the final ten days, you delete the specified food(s) as completely as possible from your diet. Suggestions—cut down on the amount of salt and salty products such as salted snacks, olives, soy sauce, processed foods, cheeses, ketchups, pickles, and yeast extracts you use. Do not use salt substitutes. Gradually reduce the number of days on which you use wheat and caffeine. Use non-wheat substitutes such as oat cakes or rye bread and crackers for wheat products and corn or buckwheat pasta for wheat pasta. Substitute non-caffeine and decaffeinated products, juices, herb, and coffee substitutes for caffeine drinks. Reduce the number of days you use alcohol and substitute non- or low-alcohol alternatives.

Using Your Muscles for Reducing Fluids

- **Walking** Find a suitable route where you will be happy to walk. Walk at a moderate speed only. Form and distance are more important than speed. Keep your body erect, your head up, and your arms slightly bent and swinging easily, but not like a march. Feel yourself relaxing and stretching into a good striding pattern. Do not carry anything in your hands and walk without any plan other than to exercise—don't use your exercise to do another chore such as shopping. Walk purposefully. Repeat your affirmation to the cadence of your walking. Run the film! Smile your "success" smile!

- **Virtual Skipping** This is skipping or jumping rope without the rope. Just let your imagination take over and think about what children and boxers do with a skipping rope—except you can't get it tangled in your feet. Remember to use your arms and wrists to twirl the imaginary rope and jump or skip on the spot, on one or both feet, using any and all the fancy combinations or elaborations you can imagine. Have fun!

- **Virtual Hula Hoop** This is just what it sounds like. Pretend you are spinning a hula hoop around and around your hips and waist just as you probably did when you were younger. Don't forget, the movement of your body has to be circular, or your imaginary hula hoop will end up around your ankles!

- **Special Exercises** This heading includes a variety of exercises to stimulate your body/mind process. Take as long as you need to complete the time or number of repetitions required by your schedule without overtiring or losing good form. Yours are:

❑ *Trunk Curls* Lie on your back on the floor on a soft mat or folded towel to protect the base of your spine. Bend your legs and place the soles of your feet flat on the floor. Place a small cushion between your knees and hold it there by squeezing your knees together. Put the palms of your hands alongside your ears, but do not hold your head or place your hands behind it. This is your start position. The action is to slowly pull your knees toward your chest and pull your chest down toward your knees, only so far as is comfortable and without straining. Don't forget to keep hold of the pillow between your knees. At maximum "curl" hold for three seconds, then stretch back to your start position and relax. Repeat as many times as required by your schedule.

- ❑ *Outer Leg Raises* Lie on your side on your mat or towel to protect the hip you are resting on. You now have a top and bottom leg and a top and bottom arm. Bend the bottom leg that's flat on the floor, keep the top leg stretched straight out, so you make a figure 4 shape with your legs. Rest the palm of your top hand on the floor in front of your chest and stretch your bottom arm out to cradle your head. You should now be in a stable position on your side. This is your start position. The action is to raise the top, outstretched leg slowly as far as it will comfortably go. Hold for three seconds and slowly lower it to the start position. Relax. Repeat as many times as required by your schedule. Turn over onto your other side and assume the start position. Repeat the exercise this way as many times as required by your schedule.

- **Your Choice Exercises** There is a space in your Strategy for you to write in and record your own exercise preferences, should you already exercise regularly. If you do, you might want to try something different. Your body soon adapts to what it is used to and fails to get the same benefits from your usual exercises. Try distance swimming (that's real swimming with proper form, which means getting your head and face in the water), rebounding, yoga, or tai chi. Heavy exercises such as weights and aerobics are useful for driving fluid from the body, provided you build up gradually to a safe level.

- **Rest Days** These are days in your schedule when you do not exercise so your body can assimilate what you've done and can deal with accumulated toxins in your muscles.

Safety Tip: To test that you are working to the right level, make certain that you can talk or sing with just a *hint* of breathlessness while you exercise. Exerting yourself to that point and no further is an easy-to-measure guide to keep you within safe limits. If you cannot talk or sing while you exercise, stop or slow down! Special note: be sure to wear good-purpose shoes such as trainers for your exercises.

Your Mind over Your Matter

- **Visualization** Check here when you've completed your visualization exercise and have a full-color, action-packed film you can run whenever you like ❑
- **Affirmation** Check here when you have created your own affirmation or have learned the affirmation provided for this Strategy and written it on each ten-day schedule in the box provided ❑

> My suggestion: "Every day little by little I RELEASE the excess WATER from my body."

(See earlier guidelines, on using your affirmation to best effect.)

Follow your daily Fluid Reduction Schedule by looking at the instructions in the column for each day and give yourself a check when you've completed them. For example, "Reduce Salt Intake by Half"— when you've done it, give yourself a check, and so on until you've completed the last day. If you have any questions refer back to the guidelines and instructions.

FLUID REDUCTION DAYS 1–10

	1	2	3	4	5	6	7	8	9	10
Eating										
Reduce salt intake by half	❑	❑	❑	❑	❑	❑	❑	❑	❑	❑
Reduce wheat intake by half	❑	❑	❑	❑	❑	❑	❑	❑	❑	❑
Reduce caffeine intake by half	❑	❑	❑	❑	❑	❑	❑	❑	❑	❑
Reduce alcohol intake by half	❑	❑	❑	❑	❑	❑	❑	❑	❑	❑
High-water day	■	■	❑	■	■	❑	■	■	❑	■
Low-water day	■	■	■	❑	■	■	❑	■	■	❑
Exercise										
Walking (10 minutes)	❑	❑	❑	■	❑	❑	❑	■	❑	❑
Virtual skipping (2 minutes)	❑	❑	❑	■	❑	❑	❑	■	❑	❑
Virtual hula hoop (30 secs each way)	❑	❑	❑	■	❑	❑	❑	■	❑	❑
Trunk curls (10 times)	❑	❑	❑	■	❑	❑	❑	■	❑	❑
Outer leg raises (6 each side)	❑	❑	❑	■	❑	❑	❑	■	❑	❑
Exercise										
Choice of exercises	❑	❑	❑	■	❑	❑	❑	■	❑	❑
Rest day	■	■	■	❑	■	■	■	❑	■	■
Mind over Matter										
Write your affirmation here:										
Affirmation (write/ say 10 times)	❑	❑	❑	❑	❑	❑	❑	❑	❑	❑

Check each box when you've completed the assignment to which it refers.

FLUID REDUCTION DAYS 11–20

	11	12	13	14	15	16	17	18	19	20
Eating										
Reduce salt intake by half again	□	□	□	□	□	□	□	□	□	□
Reduce wheat intake by half again	□	□	□	□	□	□	□	□	□	□
Reduce caffeine intake by half again	□	□	□	□	□	□	□	□	□	□
Reduce alcohol intake by half again	□	□	□	□	□	□	□	□	□	□
High-water day	■	■	■	□	■	■	■	■	□	■
Low-water day	■	■	■	■	□	■	■	■	■	□
Exercise										
Walking (15 minutes)	□	□	□	□	■	□	□	□	□	□
Virtual skipping (4 minutes)	□	□	□	□	■	□	□	□	□	□
Virtual hula hoop (60 secs each way)	□	□	□	□	■	□	□	□	□	□
Trunk curls (15 times)	□	□	□	□	■	□	□	□	□	□
Outer leg raises (9 each side)	□	□	□	□	■	□	□	□	□	□
Choice of exercises	□	□	□	□	■	□	□	□	□	□
Rest day	■	■	■	■	□	■	■	■	■	■
Mind over Matter										
Write your affirmation here:										
Affirmation (write/ say 10 times)	□	□	□	□	□	□	□	□	□	□

Check each box when you've completed the assignment to which it refers.

FLUID REDUCTION DAYS 21–30

	21	22	23	24	25	26	27	28	29	30
Eating										
Delete as much salt as you can	❑	❑	❑	❑	❑	❑	❑	❑	❑	❑
Delete as much wheat as you can	❑	❑	❑	❑	❑	❑	❑	❑	❑	❑
Delete as much caffeine as you can	❑	❑	❑	❑	❑	❑	❑	❑	❑	❑
Delete as much alcohol as you can	❑	❑	❑	❑	❑	❑	❑	❑	❑	❑
Exercise										
Walking (20 minutes)	■	❑	❑	❑	❑	❑	❑	❑	❑	■
Virtual skipping (6 minutes)	■	❑	❑	❑	❑	❑	❑	❑	❑	■
Virtual hula hoop (90 secs each way)	■	❑	❑	❑	❑	❑	❑	❑	❑	■
Trunk curls (20 times)	■	❑	❑	❑	❑	❑	❑	❑	❑	■
Outer leg raises (12 each side)	■	❑	❑	❑	❑	❑	❑	❑	❑	■
Choice of exercises	■	❑	❑	❑	❑	❑	❑	❑	❑	■
Rest day	❑	■	■	■	■	■	■	■	■	❑
Mind over Matter										
Write your affirmation here:										
Affirmation (write/ say 10 times)	❑	❑	❑	❑	❑	❑	❑	❑	❑	❑

Check each box when you've completed the assignment to which it refers.

Weight and Size Progress Chart

Weigh and measure yourself first thing on the mornings shown before any food or drink. Make sure you measure in the same place at each location on your body.

Day	1	4	7	11	14	17	21	25	28	30
Weight										
Neck										
Bust/Chest										
Waist										
Hips										
Buttocks										

THE MUSCLE RESHAPING STRATEGY

Your body has adopted an approach to eating and exercise in which general toxicity is likely to be a major part of your muscle problem, as well as adversely affecting your attitude to health and exercise. You need to alter the patterns you have created so that your system can experience functioning with fewer toxins. Your schedule shows occasional Detox days when you should eat only light meals of fruits, salads, vegetables, and rice, with water and juices as your fluids. I suggest you use the Five-Day Menu Arranger form (page 90) to plan a Detox Day menu you can use when it is needed. It might look something like this:

DETOX MENU

P = Protein, C = Carbohydrate Foods
M/A = Mix with Any, F = Fruit

	Option A	Option B
BREAKFAST	Stewed mixed fruit with flaxseeds (F)	Variety of fresh fruits with oat bran (F)
	Choose drinks from fresh fruit or vegetable juice, herb or fruit teas, and still mineral water	
	Between meals drink at least one liter of fluids from the choices offered at breakfast	
LUNCH	Green leaf salad with lemon juice and olive oil dressing (M/A)	Gazpacho (M/A)
	Steamed mixed veg on brown rice with fresh tomato sauce (C)	Large salad of mixed leaves, cucumber, beet, and raw veg with lemon juice and nut oil (M/A)
	Drink vegetable juice, herb or fruit teas	
	Between meals drink at least one liter of fluids from the choices offered at breakfast	
DINNER	Mixed salad with lemon juice and oil (M/A)	Shredded veg crudités with fresh tomato sauce (M/A)
	Steamed white fish on a bed of herbed ribbon vegetables (P)	Roast red pepper stuffed with brown rice, diced veg, and herbs (C)
	Drink vegetable juice, herb or fruit teas	
Your 1 in 5 Foods	Brown rice White fish	Brown rice Oat bran

Your Muscle Reshaping Strategy is in the form of a detailed schedule on which you will record your daily progress. Here are the instructions, guidelines, and explanations of the terms used in your Muscle Reshaping Strategy.

Muscle Reshaping Strategy—
Vital Planning Points

- Use the Five-Day Menu Arranger (page 90) to plan your eating for each day, making sure you follow the strategy outlined for the day on the Muscle Reshaping schedule above.
- **Always!** Follow strict food-combining rules (see page 43) and basic 1 in 5 food rotation. Maintain a high fluid intake— drink at least two liters of fluids per day.
- **Reduce!** Alcohol, wheat, caffeine. Reduce by half means you should aim to reduce your average daily intake in the first ten days to approximately half your previous daily average intake of the specified food. In the second ten days you should aim for a further reduction, again halving your daily intake so that it is approximately one-quarter your initial intake. The goal is to gradually reduce your intake until, in the final ten days, you delete the specified food(s) as completely as possible from your diet. Suggestions: gradually reduce the number of days on which you use wheat and caffeine. Use non-wheat substitutes such as oat crackers or rye bread and crackers for wheat products and corn or buckwheat pasta for wheat pasta. Substitute non-caffeine and decaffeinated products, juices, herb and coffee substitutes for caffeine drinks. Reduce the number of days you use alcohol and substitute non- or low-alcohol alternatives.
- **Use!** Fruit and/or stewed fruit breakfasts with flaxseed or oat bran. Brown rice, fresh fruit, vegetables and salads including raw vegetables, particularly beets. Fish, nuts and poultry in preference to red meat and dairy products.

Reshaping Your Muscles

Special notes: No limits have been allocated to the walking time in your schedule because it's assumed you'll be walking as often as you can. In fact, when using the Muscle Reshaping Strategy, you should aim to use your body as much as possible. Try the obvious first, such as walking or cycling as often as you can instead of using transport, carry your groceries from the shops, and use stairs instead of elevators. As well as increasing your overall activity and use of your body, you must develop and maintain good posture when walking, standing, or sitting. Take time to be aware, when walking, that your shoulders are relaxed, your chin is up, and your eyes are looking straight ahead, not down at your feet. Tuck your buttocks in under your spine by relaxing and straightening your lower back. Check your seats and chairs to be sure they are as comfortable as you can make them while sitting upright and relaxed. All of these small attentions will create a more complete awareness and use of your muscles, which will set you on your way. Be sure to wear good-purpose shoes such as trainers for your walking and exercises.

- **Virtual Hula Hoop** See page 138.
- **Spot Marching** Stand with your arms by your sides, chin up, and looking ahead with feet slightly apart. This is your start position. The action is to march at a medium pace, on the spot, with exaggerated arm and leg movements. Raise your knees as high as possible and your opposite arm, bent at the elbow, up as far as it will comfortably go. It really is tin soldier stuff. Continue for as long as is required by your schedule.
- **Special Exercises** This heading includes a variety of exercises to stimulate your body/mind process. Take as long as you need to complete the time or number of repetitions required by your schedule without overtiring or losing good form. Yours are:

❑ *Abdominal Contraction* See page 130.
❑ *Inner Thigh Stretch* Lie flat on your back on a small mat or folded towel to protect your back. Pull your knees up and

allow your legs to open out until you can place the soles of your feet together. Allow your knees to fall open, keeping your soles together and pulled as close to your tailbone as possible while still being comfortable. The important thing here is to allow gravity to act, so relax as completely as you can; don't force your legs apart or your knees down. Success comes from becoming conscious of the tension that keeps your inner thighs taut, then gradually letting that tension go. Stay in the "open" position for as long as is required by your schedule.

❑ *Relax* Start by lying flat on your back on the same small mat or folded towel you used for your Inner Thigh Stretch. This time lie out flat with your arms on the floor at your sides, palms up and about a foot away from your body. Your legs should be flat on the floor and your feet about shoulder-width apart. Put a thin pillow under your head to support it at a natural angle, not tipped up or back. Now close your eyes and relax; breathe deeply in and out ten times. There is nothing else to do but notice and release any tightness and tension in your body for as long as is required by your schedule—or until you wake up. Concentrate on your breathing and use the time to practice and reinforce your visualization. Run the film! Smile your "success" smile!

• **Your Choice Exercises** There is a space in your Strategy for you to write in and record your own exercise preferences, should you already exercise regularly.

• **Rest days** These are days in your schedule when you do not exercise so your body can assimilate what you've done and can deal with accumulated toxins in your muscles.

Safety Tip: To test that you are working to the right level, make certain that you can talk or sing with just a *hint* of breathlessness while you exercise. Exerting yourself to that point and no further is an easy-to-measure guide to keep you within safe limits. If you cannot talk or sing while you exercise, stop or slow down!

Your Mind over Your Matter

- **Visualization** Check here when you've completed your visualization exercise and have a full-color, action-packed film you can run whenever you like. ❑
- **Affirmation** Check here when you have created your own affirmation or have learned the affirmation provided for this Strategy and written it on each ten-day schedule in the box provided ❑

> My suggestion: "Every day little by little my MUSCLES are stronger and more toned."

(See earlier guidelines on using your affirmation to best effect.)

Follow your daily Muscle Reshaping Schedules by looking at the instructions in the column for each day, and give yourself a check when you've completed them. For example, "Reduce Alcohol Intake by Half"—when you've done it, give yourself a check, and so on until you've completed the last day. If you have any questions, refer back to the guidelines and instructions.

MUSCLE RESHAPING DAYS 1–10

	1	2	3	4	5	6	7	8	9	10
Eating										
Reduce alcohol intake by half	☐	☐	☐	☐	☐	☐	☐	☐	☐	☐
Reduce wheat intake by half	☐	☐	☐	☐	☐	☐	☐	☐	☐	☐
Reduce caffeine intake by half	☐	☐	☐	☐	☐	☐	☐	☐	☐	☐
Detox day	■	■	■	☐	■	■	■	■	☐	■
Exercise										
Virtual hula hoop (60 secs each way)	☐	☐	☐	■	☐	☐	☐	■	☐	☐
Spot marching (2 minutes)	☐	☐	☐	■	☐	☐	☐	■	☐	☐
Abdominal contraction (8 times)	☐	☐	☐	■	☐	☐	☐	■	☐	☐
Inner thigh stretch (1 minute)	☐	☐	☐	■	☐	☐	☐	■	☐	☐
Relax (2 minutes)	☐	☐	☐	■	☐	☐	☐	■	☐	☐
Choice of exercises	☐	☐	☐	■	☐	☐	☐	■	☐	☐
Rest day	■	■	■	☐	■	■	■	☐	■	■
Mind over Matter										
Write your affirmation here:										
Affirmation (write/ say 10 times)	☐	☐	☐	☐	☐	☐	☐	☐	☐	☐

Check each box when you've completed the assignment to which it refers.

MUSCLE RESHAPING DAYS 11–20

	11	12	13	14	15	16	17	18	19	20
Eating										
Reduce alcohol intake by half again	❑	❑	❑	❑	❑	❑	❑	❑	❑	❑
Reduce wheat intake by half again	❑	❑	❑	❑	❑	❑	❑	❑	❑	❑
Reduce caffeine intake by half again	❑	❑	❑	❑	❑	❑	❑	❑	❑	❑
Detox day	■	■	■	❑	■	■	■	■	❑	■
Exercise										
Virtual hula hoop (90 secs each way)	❑	❑	❑	❑	■	❑	❑	❑	❑	❑
Spot marching (3 minutes)	❑	❑	❑	❑	■	❑	❑	❑	❑	❑
Abdominal contraction (12 times)	❑	❑	❑	❑	■	❑	❑	❑	❑	❑
Inner thigh stretch (2 minutes)	❑	❑	❑	❑	■	❑	❑	❑	❑	❑
Relax (3 minutes)	❑	❑	❑	❑	■	❑	❑	❑	❑	❑
Choice of exercises	❑	❑	❑	❑	■	❑	❑	❑	❑	❑
Rest day	■	■	■	■	❑	■	■	■	■	■
Mind over Matter										
Write your affirmation here:										
Affirmation (write/ say 10 times)	❑	❑	❑	❑	❑	❑	❑	❑	❑	❑

Check each box when you've completed the assignment to which it refers.

MUSCLE RESHAPING DAYS 21–30

	21	22	23	24	25	26	27	28	29	30
Eating										
Delete as much alcohol as you can	□	□	□	□	□	□	□	□	□	□
Delete as much wheat as you can	□	□	□	□	□	□	□	□	□	□
Delete as much caffeine as you can	□	□	□	□	□	□	□	□	□	□
Detox day	■	■	■	□	■	■	■	■	□	■
Exercise										
Virtual hula hoop (2 mins each way)	■	□	□	□	□	□	□	□	□	■
Spot marching (4 minutes)	■	□	□	□	□	□	□	□	□	■
Abdominal contraction (16 times)	■	□	□	□	□	□	□	□	□	■
Inner thigh stretch (3 minutes)	■	□	□	□	□	□	□	□	□	■
Relax (5 minutes)	■	□	□	□	□	□	□	□	□	■
Choice of exercises	■	□	□	□	□	□	□	□	□	■
Rest day	□	■	■	■	■	■	■	■	■	□
Mind over Matter										
Write your affirmation here:										
Affirmation (write/ say 10 times)	□	□	□	□	□	□	□	□	□	□

Check each box when you've completed the assignment to which it refers.

Weight and Size Progress Chart

Weigh and measure yourself first thing on the mornings shown before any food or drink. Make sure you measure in the same place at each location on your body.

Day	1	4	7	11	14	17	21	25	28	30
Weight										
Neck										
Bust/Chest										
Waist										
Hips										
Buttocks										

CONGRATULATIONS!

You ought to be really proud of yourself for what you've just achieved. It doesn't matter whether you completed all thirty days perfectly or managed only a part of what was suggested for you in your Strategy; you've already accomplished a great deal.

In thirty days you've made a major adjustment. You've changed your body and altered the ways you think and feel about yourself. You've learned even more about what makes you the way you are and how you can improve yourself. And you've established a new foundation from which you can go forward to even greater improvements, if you want to.

It is your personal strength, spirit, and commitment which has enabled you to accomplish all that you have already. And these same rather rare qualities will help you progress further still.

So is it enough? Are you fully satisfied with your body yet? The answer is probably "No!"

First of all, thirty days, no matter how transforming, is not enough to restore the effects of a lifelong process that has been working in some quite inappropriate ways. You're not likely to have achieved all you can or all you want, yet. Clearly this is not the end of the story. The question now has to be: What next?

Well, your eating is *under control*. Food combining is second nature to you now. During your Strategy you've dramatically reduced your intake of certain foods which are keys to your weight, shape, and health. It will take very little effort for you to keep your intake of those foods down to a minimum or make them, at most, 1 in 5. Also, during the past thirty days you've made exercise a part of your normal routine. That's the hard part, and to continue exercising now will be much easier for you.

A good idea would be for you to return now to basic Kensington Way eating and add what you've learned about your eating and exercise from the Strategy you've just completed. In fact, I expect you'll find it hard to do otherwise, because you'll feel uncomfortable with your old, bad eating habits.

If you want to pursue still further improvements, you might, at some appropriate time soon, repeat the Strategy you've just done, or you might prefer to use one of the other Strategies if it seems more relevant. You may even use your new knowledge and self-understanding to create a special program—just for yourself.

Whatever you choose to do, you need to consider the long term. You will maintain a body shape, weight, and state of health commensurate with the level of regular self-care you sustain.

Occasional, powerful short-term strategies are useful for major changes to your situation. You can't, however, expect to keep the improvements you've made, let alone improve further, if you don't make these essentials—good eating, good exercise, and good thinking—intrinsic with your way of life.

I don't believe you can be successful if these essentials are chores you have to struggle to do on a regular basis. Self-care has to become pleasurable, exciting, fun, and as natural a part of your healthy life as your old bad habits were to your unhealthy one.

I hope you have already realized, from your experiences so far with *Love Food . . . Lose Weight* and your slimming Strategy that it's entirely possible to achieve that goal.

Anything more extreme than you are able to do regularly with the minimum of effort and disruption to the lifestyle you enjoy most is likely to fail in the final analysis. If you embark upon major distortions of eating and lifestyle, you'll soon find yourself where you once were—oscillating between drastic health or weight cures and old bad habits. It shows a lack of self-understanding and will send you back into the old spiral of health and weight crises—the same old story of perpetual crisis management to wrench you back from the brink of obesity while your health deteriorates ever downward.

The answer to the question "What's next?" then, is to choose a level of self-care that you can enjoy and stick to. If you do so, you'll achieve and maintain your best Appropriate Body—that is, the size, weight, and level of health consistent with the best self-image you can achieve and most healthy lifestyle that you are willing to commit to and can enjoy.

In short, you need to learn to live the good life *that's good for you*. The next chapter will help you discover how to make your good life as good as it can be.

CHAPTER

5

A Better-Body Lifestyle

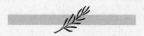

THE GOOD LIFE THAT'S GOOD FOR YOU!

Here's a promise from me to you. When you incorporate the *Love Food . . . Lose Weight* diet into your everyday life, you'll find you are enjoying your life more than ever, while your body gets better and better.

You won't have to pursue the impossible goal of keeping to an austere regime of diet and exercise. You'll be able to *enjoy* fantastic food and do only the exercise you want. You won't have to worry that the practicalities of modern living will overtake your good intentions to be healthy and slim. You won't become an antisocial health freak or a slimming bore! And you will almost certainly wonder why you didn't start caring for yourself this way sooner.

One of the many reasons most diets and health improvement systems fail is that they make no distinction between the strict regimes and disciplines that quickly get your weight and health under control, and strategies required for *maintaining* the improvements you made.

You and I know that what you are able to do for short periods to improve your health and dimensions is far and away from what you can continue to do in your normal busy life. Inevitably, even your best efforts to continue with strict eating programs and exercise regimes are going to be overcome by the demands of day-to-day living in the modern world.

What about entertaining? What happens when you want to eat out? What if you want to continue to eat properly but your partner or children will not? What happens if you break the rules? Can you recover lost ground if you eat a "bad" meal? How much time do you have to spend on exercise?

These are practical considerations to take into account when fitting self-care into everyday living. They require a different approach from the intensive methods you can employ during the first few short weeks of a new health program. Your initial flush of enthusiasm will carry you through the disruption of daily life early on, but what happens when you have to get back to the real world?

The *Love Food . . . Lose Weight* diet is set apart from other diets and health systems by one feature more than any other: the ease with which *it* can adapt to fit into *your* lifestyle, so your life just keeps on getting better.

The *Love Food . . . Lose Weight* diet works with, not against, the ever-changing process that is behind your health, your shape, and your life experience. It works not by assuming you can be fixed perpetually in some state of "healthy" or "not fat," but by recognizing your body, mind, and life are all in a constant state of adjustment and alteration that can be guided. The *Love Food . . . Lose Weight* diet works because it prompts and supports changes in your body and mind that mean your health and figure will gradually improve rather than deteriorate.

The continuous processing that is the ecology of your body and mind cannot stand still. You will and *must* continue to change—it's part of the experience of being alive. Permanent good health and long-term weight control demand that you change in positive, health-giving ways. You must establish and maintain a *momentum for improvement*.

The key to successfully incorporating self-care into your everyday life is this: *support the process* of beneficial change at a worthwhile level—one you can enjoy and accommodate.

The methods you've used so far in this diet have had a threefold purpose. First, to provide you with as much benefit to your health and shape as possible in a short time. Second, to help you acquire the basic principles of self-care. Third, and probably the most important, to redirect the process that underpins all that you are, and set it on a firm foundation for further improvement.

Once you've established a momentum for improvement, you can

relax considerably from constant attention to your health and shape. As long as you are practicing a reasonable degree of self-care most of the time, the evolving process of your body/mind will continue to bring about improvements, and you need not worry about slipping back.

The basic *Love Food . . . Lose Weight* way of eating taught you the simple ground rules, and huge benefits can be gained, in health and weight, from staying *as close as possible* to these guidelines. However, provided that—*most* of the time (say 80 percent)—you combine your food correctly and rotate foods which cause you a problem, it won't hurt you to bend the rules occasionally, especially if you know how to do it and *still* benefit! So here I present you with some "street-smart" eating advice, some diet tricks that have come from many years' experience, some new ways of looking at what's healthy and what's not.

How to Bend the Rules and Still Benefit

Purist food combiners are going to hate this, but the truth is that there's more than a little wisdom in the saying "Rules are made to be broken." I know from many years of direct experience—not textbook theorizing—that you *can* bend good eating rules and get away with it. In fact, you'll find that it can actually be *good* for you to occasionally break the rules! Let me explain.

The vastly complex system that is your body/mind has specifically evolved to deal with and overcome difficulties and problems. You are a problem-solving organism, one which *thrives* on rising to meet a challenge—as long as that problem *is capable of* being solved and doesn't persist too long.

A meal that doesn't conform to your good eating ideals presents your body with a *challenge*. Therefore, the occasional meal outside guidelines can actually be used to stimulate your body to *greater efficiency*. In other words, "bad" eating can sometimes be good for you!

What you need to understand is this: you can *sometimes* bend the rules *only* when you are otherwise keeping to them most of the time. It's important not to let things get out of hand. And when you *do* bend the rules, you must bend them to your advantage. Let's take another look at the guidelines, and I'll show you what I mean.

The main food-combining rule is: Eat Proteins and Carbohydrates so they won't be in your stomach at the same time. Another rule is to eat fruits on their own or only with other fruits.

Now, these two rules pose a challenge if you want to serve a sweet dessert after any meal and stay within the food-combining rules. Clearly you shouldn't serve a dessert containing starchy carbohydrates like rice or wheat after a protein meal. The opposite is also true—you shouldn't serve protein-rich desserts such as ice cream, eggs, or yogurt after a starchy meal. And since many desserts contain fruit, they ought not be served after either protein or starchy foods. So if you want to eat something sweet after a meal, what can you do?

Here are some suggestions. They're not the best combinations, but they'll be much better for you than reaching for chocolate pudding after roast chicken.

Let's deal with the easy one first: what to have after carbohydrate/ starchy meals, such as pasta, rice or potatoes. Both sugars and high-starch foods are carbohydrates, so a sweet and starchy dessert after a starch meal is not a bad combination. So far no problem, except you can't expect that sort of meal to be helpful to your weight if you eat it too often.

Fruit is not advised as a dessert at any meal, carbohydrate or protein, because fruits pass quickly through your stomach to be digested very rapidly elsewhere in your digestive system. If you mix fruits with foods that need longer in your stomach or intestines they may have time to ferment, or they may disrupt your digestion and disturb your digestive environment in some other way.

However . . . *some* fruits are so high in sugars they can virtually be described as carbohydrates. So, if after a starchy meal you want a dessert, you could have fruit as long as it's *very* sweet fruit. I suggest you have sweet ripe fruits with cream (which is a Mix With Any food), or fruit sorbets, flans, or pies. The sweetest fruits are dried fruits, because their sugars have been concentrated by drying.

What about sweet desserts after protein meals? According to the rules, fruits would not be a good idea. But . . . *some* fruits contain enzymes which actually help in the digestion of animal proteins. So, after a protein meal you could reasonably make a dessert from papaya, mango, ripe bananas, pineapple, or apples. Use them in sorbets or on their own. With or without cream, depending on the role of high-fat foods in your diet.

One of the main reasons carbohydrate/protein combining is regarded as a problem is because starches are not efficiently broken down in a digestive environment needed to deal with proteins. But while that's true for starch carbohydrates, it's not necessarily true for sugar carbohydrates—the conversion of which is not affected in the same way. This gives you more latitude for sweet desserts after protein meals when, as Winnie the Pooh says, it's "time for something sweet"!

Some delicious sugar/protein combinations make classic desserts. Sugar and eggs = zabaglione, crème caramel, crème brûlée or chocolate mousse; sugar and dairy = ice cream or yogurt with honey and nuts.

A warning here: I'm making suggestions for *very occasional* relaxations of your regular good eating habits. Sugar/protein combining has a major pitfall in connection with your weight and shape. Many proteins are *high-fat* foods. Desserts often require a high fat content. Fatty foods mixed with carbohydrates, particularly sugar-rich carbohydrates, ought to be avoided if you're trying to reduce body fat.

So bend the rules like this if you want to—from time to time—but also understand that the desire for something sweet after a meal is more often a desire for a taste to balance and clear the palate, not for more food to fill space left after one or two earlier courses.

So, instead of making a big, rich dessert course after a meal, why not accommodate the need for something sweet after either protein or starch meals with a light sorbet of coffee, chocolate, or mint? You could even sweeten up something that's usually savory. A wealthy client of mine who ate at many of the best restaurants in the world frequently asked for a salad with a *sweet vinaigrette* to end her meal. That's a vinaigrette made with rather more honey than usual, or perhaps with a sweet vinegar.

My favorite solution is to make a substantial meal of well-combined early courses and please my palate with a couple of good-quality chocolates and an exquisite dessert wine. Who could resist and what digestive system would complain?

The rules of food rotating can be relaxed as well, although at first it seems to be more complicated to do.

The food rotation rule, you'll recall, is:

All proteins, carbohydrates, and foods liable to be eaten very often—other than vegetables, salads, and fruits—should be eaten one day only in any five days.

Food rotating varies your diet for a particularly important reason. Some foods, if eaten too often, can seriously affect your health or figure. At the very least, rotating means you're going to avoid a high intake of potentially troublesome foods. At best, you'll be able to identify and remove from your diet foods that have already become a problem for you.

In fact, among the list of 1 in 5 foods there are only a few that are often found to be troublesome. They are wheat, potatoes, and sugars amongst the carbohydrates, eggs, cow's dairy products (especially cheese), caffeine products, chocolate, and soy. Let's call them the *high-risk* 1 in 5's.

Most of the remaining foods on the list are proteins, for which strict 1 in 5 rotation may be desirable but is not *always* essential. They are *low-risk* 1 in 5 foods. As long as you take care to avoid frequent use of any particular protein, you can occasionally eat whatever protein you want with less than the recommended four days between servings.

So there's no need to upset Aunty Mabel if you visit and she serves you salmon for dinner when you had salmon the previous day. Enjoy it! It's unlikely, after all, that you'll choose salmon again tomorrow or even within the next few days.

However, when bending the rules for high-risk 1 in 5 foods, you need to take more care. These foods are more likely to cause you problems if you overuse them. They're also most likely to have been habit foods which you've used too often in the past.

If you reintroduce into your diet a large or frequent intake of foods you've managed to reduce to 1 in 5, you run the risk they will quickly become reestablished as habit foods, with all the unpleasant consequences that entails.

There is a way to ease the restrictions around the short list of high-risk 1 in 5 foods.

When you've identified the foods you have overused in the past, make them as scarce in your diet as possible by reducing your intake to *even less* than 1 in 5. If then, on a rare occasion, you do eat any of them, you're not likely to have any lasting problems. You'll be able to thoroughly enjoy the food as an unaccustomed treat. This applies mainly to problem carbohydrates such as wheat and potatoes, and also cheese, soy, eggs, and chocolate.

You won't be able to do this so easily with foods like milk, sugar, and salt. These are items you may have identified from your Slimming Strategy as being involved with your weight or health. You've probably already reduced them to very small amounts in your diet. You may even have deleted them altogether.

Remember, when you decide how much to relax the rules for these foods, you are deciding what *compromises* you are prepared to make with your health and shape. You may decide that regular but small amounts of milk, sugar, or salt affect you only marginally, and you are prepared to put up with their minor ill effects. Only you can know and choose. My advice is to bring these foods completely under control and experience what you feel like without them, *then* make your "compromise" decision. The gradual reduction method in the weight-control Strategies shows you how.

This is particularly true for one of the most powerful social drugs in the world, caffeine. If you have not been caffeine-free since your teens or earlier, when you started drinking cola, tea, and coffee, you'd be wise to clean it from your system and find out how it's been affecting you. Then decide how to use it in future.

My advice is to use caffeine no more than 1 in 5 and stick as rigidly to that discipline as you possibly can. Only if you are totally confident in your ability to bring your caffeine intake under control should you bend that rule. At all other times, I believe the health penalties from decaffeinated products are far preferable to those of frequent caffeine use, and you should use decaffeinated products or alternative hot drinks.

When only one day in five is a caffeine day, it can become a useful but not essential item in your momentum for health. When you use caffeine periodically, it gives occasional stimulation to your brain and several systems in your body. It can act as an intermittent diuretic and laxative and a prompt to your metabolism, for example.

That's *not* what happens if you use caffeine so frequently that you become habituated to it. If your body is being constantly driven by a high and probably increasing caffeine intake, your mental and physical functions are becoming reliant on the drug and are *losing their capacity* to function well without it.

There is one final way you can relax the good eating rules you've acquired through the *Love Food . . . Lose Weight* diet and your Strategies. That is to let them go entirely!

All your efforts to date will not be destroyed if on rare occasions you eat a meal that *totally* ignores all the rules. For the reasons I've already explained, it may even be good for you.

It is not good for a dynamic, developing organism such as you are to be restricted to rigid habits—no matter how beneficial they are supposed to be. It's good to walk on the wild side of your diet sometimes.

The key issue is not whether you bend or break the rules, but if you can use the occasions on which you do for your *benefit.* I've explained how rare incidents of bad eating can stimulate your body functions. Those episodes can also be used to reinforce your self-image and your intent to become healthier and slimmer.

Strict dieting through guilt, shame, frustration, or anger will not work in the long term. Compassionate self-care must be at the core of your healthy eating.

One way of demonstrating your compassion and self-care is by being able to give yourself *permission* to bend the rules when it is safe and appropriate to do so. There are many other ways in which you can demonstrate self-care with your food. One way is by *imposing* rules on yourself; another is by *relaxation* of the same rules. It will depend on the circumstances and your motives on the occasion, whether your choice is self-enabling or self-defeating. Only you will be able to tell.

My sincere advice is: "Everything right most of the time, most things right all of the time, and a few things wrong some of the time." Follow that and you'll always be healthy and in good shape.

IN CASE OF DIET EMERGENCY— THINK 10 PERCENT!

If at any time you need to improve your control of your health or dimensions, the basic *Love Food . . . Lose Weight* diet and your chosen Strategy offer a wealth of resources on which to fall back. All you have to do to reestablish good habits is to return to the techniques and helpful tips you've already used. To speed up progress where you may have become lax or lost momentum, simply create for yourself a short strategy from those methods you now know will work the best for you. For example, you can return to strict food combining for a week, and reduce your intake of a food you think is not helping to keep your weight under control. After a few days of eating rich food, you can turn to a day or two of detox eating, as described in chapter 4 (page 145). These techniques can now be used at your convenience. All the methods you've acquired can be fitted into your schedule as and when *you* choose.

If you are not ready to start a thirty-day Strategy, here's a way to start getting your weight and shape under control—fast!

The 10 Percent Rule is simplicity itself. All you have to do is *reduce* your intake of proteins, carbohydrates, and fats by 10 percent and *increase* your physical activity by—you've got it—10 percent. Of course, you must carry on your good food combining and 1 in 5 food rotations at the same time.

This straightforward adjustment to your established eating/activity ratio can bring about a major shift in your metabolism. You'll be responding to the demands of more activity with less food by using the fuel available from your food better and not wasting (or waisting!) it as excess fat on your body.

Here are a few tips:

- Use 10 percent more stairs, even if you have to retrace your steps a little.
- Walk 10 percent more than you do now, even if you have to take the long cut rather than the shortcut.
- Make love 10 percent more, dig a tenth of the garden over twice, take the dog for that extra walk, and so on.

And when you are ready to eat, simply use a plate that's 10 percent smaller or prepare 10 percent less in the first place. If you are still hungry, steam some vegetables or make a salad and dress them with a squeeze of lemon juice and some freshly ground black pepper. As a last resort, donate 10 percent to the dog or the dustbin and think of it not as waste but as an investment in your waist.

The 10 Percent Rule really is your emergency button, for it accomplishes quickly and with little effort a true paring down in your food and your figure, and prepares you for a lengthier, more detailed approach when the time is right.

EATING AT HOME AND AWAY

On some occasions it's going to be more of a challenge for you to keep to the rules than others. Here's some advice that will make it easier for you to fit the *Love Food . . . Lose Weight* diet into your home, social, and business life.

Your own home is where it's easiest to control what you eat. At home, you can make sure you have available the foods you enjoy and which can be fitted into your good eating pattern. You can keep to strict combining, rotating, and more easily control the amount you eat. You can ensure you and your family have well combined and rotated food at work or school, when you prepare it at home.

So it's at home you should establish a credit balance of good eating from which to draw on those occasions when you might choose to eat not so well. At home you can turn the debit of any bad eating into a credit, by using food wisely to restore yourself after any unhelpful meals. The main difficulties with healthy eating at home arise when catering for a family or when entertaining guests.

For example, if your partner prefers not to follow your healthy eating rules, that shouldn't cause you to abandon what you are doing for yourself. It really takes very little extra effort to create meals from which one item can be excluded or included according to the desire to follow combining rules or not.

The traditional roast is a case in point. This meal usually consists of roasted meat protein with some Mix With Any vegetables and a carbohydrate (usually roast potatoes). To make it a carbohydrate meal, leave out the meat. To make it a protein meal, leave out the potatoes. After all, if your partner didn't like one of the vegetables and preferred not to have it in their meal, you wouldn't consider it a problem; nor should it be if one of you prefers to leave out the protein or carbohydrate. Whoever cooks the meal isn't likely to find it too arduous, either, to prepare an extra vegetable or two to make up for an item that's been left out.

My mother cooks the best roast potatoes in the world! Doesn't every mother? So I eat her roast meals with meat and about five Mix With Any vegetables, and she keeps some of the potatoes for me to eat later. I could just as easily keep the protein component of the meal back and eat it cold with salad another time. It's easy, isn't it?

I know that children can be especially troublesome about what they will and won't eat. With young children you, as their parent, can direct what they will have on their plate. The sooner you start giving children well-combined food, the more likely they are to accept it. If, however, your children are used to eating poorly combined meals and they are of an age when directing their eating is not appropriate, the solution is to make flexible meals from which items can be removed—in the way I've described above. Alternatively, have meals in which the rules have been relaxed only moderately, again as I've described before.

Entertaining guests can be enjoyed with little or no compromise of your good eating habits when you extend the invitations from your own home. It's simplicity itself to create a multiple-course dinner party within *Love Food . . . Lose Weight* guidelines; just look at chapter 6 to see how. If you choose to relax the rules for guests, it will be your decision as to how much and how far you'll do so.

Eating out at restaurants doesn't have to be difficult either. The key thing to remember is you are the customer and are entitled to have your meal the way *you* want it. So, ask for what you want! Ask for information about the dishes on the menu. Explain what you need and ask for advice. It's a poor restaurant that is unable to offer some help or that cannot accommodate modest changes to their dishes.

It may be going a little too far to tell your waiter you need to alter the chef's creations in order to avoid allergic reactions, as one of my American friends suggested, but that would probably guarantee their attention! I suspect it would be better to do what I've done frequently in even the choicest eating places. Choose the main item you'd like, even though it may be shown accompanied by foods that won't mix well, then glance at what is being offered with other dishes that can replace offending items in your meal.

I recall pointing out to an increasingly excited chef how the celery root purée, offered elsewhere with pork, and the ratatouille shown accompanying a fish dish, would perfectly replace the mashed potato which was being offered with the lamb cutlets I wanted. The chef found he was creating a new dish especially for me from ingredients he already had, and was pleased to do so.

The ethnic and culinary style of the restaurant can make choices easy for you. Here are a few suggestions about the meals you could enjoy in a variety of different eating establishments.

Chinese/Thai/Other Asian

Asian cooking is great for braised or stir-fried vegetables, served on their own or with proteins or carbohydrates included in the dish. So for your diet, look for a good variety of Mix With Any vegetables, then go for the proteins or carbohydrates you want to go with them and which fit with your 1 in 5 eating plan.

Protein accompaniments can be fish, shellfish, poultry and meats, tofu and nuts, including coconut but not peanuts, which come under carbohydrates. Watch out that these options are not served wrapped in pancakes, as dim sum or wontons, deep-fried in batter, or tossed in cornstarch or similar before cooking.

Carbohydrates can be rice, of course, and don't forget rice noodles, but not egg noodles, rice pancakes, and peanuts are OK.

Italian

The Italians too know how to make vegetables exciting in a meal, so how about checking out first the many Mix With Any vegetables traditionally found in the Mediterranean area. You can expect to find puréed, roasted, sautéed, and braised vegetables mixed with garlic, herbs, and olive oil. The Italians make delicious salads as well, using a wide range of Mix With Any vegetables and salad ingredients. But remember, prefer simple dressings and leave out the Parmesan or croutons if they won't mix with the other foods you choose.

Now examine the proteins available to go with your M/A vegetables or salad. Fish and shellfish will figure strongly, as will chicken and other poultry. Also the whole range of meats and some forms of beef innards will be offered too, but make sure they're not dusted with flour prior to pan frying or coated in bread crumbs before deep frying. Perfect dishes will be found broiled, griddle-fried, or roasted.

Carbohydrate in Italy means pasta first and foremost. Which is fine for you so long as it's the non-egg pasta used by most natives of that country. You can eat it with tomato sauces, your Mix With Any vegetables, or with a whole range of herbs and other Mix With Any flavorings. Also try polenta and wonderful Italian breads and even pizza if it has loads of tomato sauce and perhaps garlic, onions, olives, and herbs but no cheese or meat protein on top.

French

Trying to categorize French cuisine is a forlorn task, the variety is so great, but here goes. You'll probably find delicious, crisp, and very lightly blanched M/A European garden vegetables, some braised varieties, and wonderful specialties like ratatouille. Also salads, but as before you'll want simple M/A ingredients and good dressings without additional proteins or carbohydrates.

To go with your choice of M/A foods, look for exquisitely cooked proteins of all varieties from fish and shellfish to poultry of all kinds and every meat available. Steer clear of quiches, tarts, and croutons, no matter how tempting, if eating proteins. French cheeses are superb and go well with crisp, clean crudités as a starter, light meal, or dessert. The delight of French cooking is it can make a memorable meal out of virtually anything.

Carbohydrate meals are risky if eating French food. Not because it can't be done, but you'll probably upset the entire staff of any French restaurant if you try to get away with just eating potatoes and vegetables, and french fries or baguette with salad just won't endear you at all.

Indian/Arabic

There is a similarity between these styles of cooking even though the spices and flavorings are so different. You can select a variety of deliciously cooked Mix With Any vegetables, then add in your choice of protein or carbohydrate. Take care the vegetables don't have curd cheese or carbohydrates like potatoes, corn, or beans if your accompanying choice is to be protein.

Proteins are delicious in both these styles of cooking, and you will find baked, roasted, and griddled meats and poultry in a variety of joints, cuts, and even on skewers.

Carbohydrate options are just as varied if not more so. Special breads are available from both countries, as are a variety of dishes which combine beans or lentils with M/A vegetables. Gram flour batters, daals, and papadoms from India are especially good or choose couscous and tabbouleh from the Middle East and put them with roasted M/A vegetables.

Mexican

The Mix With Any foods you can choose from if eating Mexican cuisine include not just vegetables and salads but wonderful salsas, avocado, especially in the form of guacamole, and sour cream, many flavored with M/A chilies. Choose from what's available and plan your meal with your selection of protein or carbohydrates to go with them.

Proteins can be fish, meat, or poultry and are best simply barbecued or broiled, or in delicious stews. Try beef with chocolate if you can get it.

Various carbohydrates are staples in Mexican cuisine, so be careful they don't infringe into protein meals; for instance, nachos with cheese won't work. Enjoy flour or corn tortillas and burritos, refried beans, corn chips, and corn kernels with the M/A vegetables and salads.

Greek/Turkish/Israeli

The M/A vegetable and salad options are as varied in these styles of cuisine as they are in other Mediterranean countries, and you can choose quite well from a good variety which reflect Middle East and Mediterranean cooking influences. Don't forget the olives and pickled peppers.

Proteins, that is, meats, poultry, and fish, are best simply grilled, roasted, or broiled. My favorite from Greece is kleftiko, a small leg joint of lamb roasted at a low heat for hours until it melts in the mouth, but not served with the traditional Greek–style roast potatoes. From Turkey I enjoy the baked and roasted sweet peppers, zucchini, and eggplants.

Carbohydrates are delicious, too, with beans used in all styles of cooking, stewed with M/A vegetables, puréed as in hummus, or formed into falafel with herbs. Pita bread goes well with salads or vegetables from any of the regions.

We often go to restaurants to eat the kinds of cuisine we don't have every day. We go to enjoy special food in special surroundings, and in those circumstances you may decide to relax the strict interpretation of your good eating rules in one or other of the ways I've explained.

If you choose to bend the rules, bend them thoughtfully. If, for example, you've been eating well for quite a while, you have wheat under control in your diet, and you're enjoying your new diet, why succumb to the inevitable bread roll offered by many restaurants before a meal? Far better to forgo the bread (ask for some crudités if you want to nibble before your meal arrives) and instead spoil yourself with a delicious dessert. You can have bread any day, but desserts in a good restaurant are to be taken advantage of! Personally, I enjoy waiting until I get to a restaurant to eat cheese, with crudités of course, because restaurants generally have a much wider variety of unusual cheeses than is practical for me to have at home.

In the last resort, you must choose how particular you want to be about your good eating rules for that restaurant meal. Whatever you decide to do, though, make up your mind quickly, stick firmly to your decision, then above all else *enjoy* the meal. Nothing is worse than eating a delicious meal in an excellent restaurant with your mind full of regrets.

When you go away on vacation, the strong sense of freedom and relaxation can make the idea of dieting seem like a wet blanket on an otherwise pleasant experience. It doesn't have to be that way. Food combining and food rotation means wherever you are, you can keep close enough to the rules that you'll still be in the same shape when you return home.

To inspire you to keep as closely as possible to your healthy eating habits, let me share a word of caution about uncontrolled vacation eating. When you've been eating well for a while, you'll respond quite severely to sudden indiscriminate combining and overuse of foods. Eat in your old, bad ways and you may enjoy the taste reward for a short while, but you *won't* enjoy how you feel afterward. The feelings of discomfort in your digestion and the shifts of mood which result can really spoil your holiday. Take a tip: enjoy your vacation, bend the rules a little, but *don't* break them.

Now let's discuss what is probably the most difficult dining situation you'll encounter. The dinner party at someone else's home. All types of catering can be found. From hosts you may know well to those you know not at all . . . from cooking that's sublime to positively lethal . . . and menus that are a joy or seem to have been concocted by Torquemada. When the modern host and hostess set out to decide on a menu, they are beset by a variety of different influences and inspirations. Generosity, or lack of it, genuine caring, hospitality, bad judgment, and plain showing off have inspired many a food-combining disaster!

At events like these we all stumble and fall over the hurdles placed before our good intentions. Here are some hard-won hints on how to keep on course with your good eating.

Talk to your hostess, especially if she's a friend. You may discover she's a committed food combiner, although I have to say that's no guarantee your meal will be well combined; sometimes even food combiners seem driven to extraordinary behavior when creating dinner party menus for guests. In any event, by talking you can explain—preferably before you show up—that you follow good combining rules whenever you can. That should preempt any frosty frowns if you are observed avoiding some items because they don't combine well. Who knows? If you have a chat beforehand, your hostess may even create a menu that makes things easy for you.

Think of it like this. Would you prefer a guest of yours to tell you about their dietary preferences before you prepared and served a meal, or would you prefer to watch as they left something and then spend the evening wondering why?

If the thought of discussing how you eat is too dire and you haven't got the nerve or willpower to leave some items, your best option is to eat all that is put before you. You can always put a recovery plan into operation tomorrow and allow the experience to be the bad that's good for you!

That may actually be your only option. It's amazing how many menus are contrived from recipes in which entirely incompatible foods are so completely mixed that you couldn't separate them with a magnifying glass and scalpel, let alone a knife and fork.

Remember, though, all of it is being perpetrated on you in the name of hospitality, so if bad food is inevitable, sit back, enjoy it with good grace, and think of tomorrow, when you can restore your equilibrium and renew your good intentions to eat healthily. Console yourself with the thought that you can't break the rules so badly that you can *never* recover.

If the food you've eaten was much richer than you are used to, your system will be stimulated to deal with it. Your gallbladder, liver, and colon in particular will get a truly valuable workout. You can help your body after a bad eating choice by eating two very simple meals, without carbohydrates or proteins, for each bad meal you've eaten. A rich and heavy meal therefore becomes the precursor to a short period of stimulation and cleansing which adds impetus to your drive for improvement. Provided such elaborate meals are not eaten too frequently!

High-calorie meals too can be used to your advantage. Give yourself a metabolism boost by following any high-calorie meal with a day of very low-calorie eating.

In either case, make your follow-up meals from lots of fruits, salads, and vegetables. Drink plenty of water and juices. If you have proteins, make them light and easy to digest—fish and chicken, for example. If you have carbohydrates, make them cleansing ones such as rice or oats.

Believe me, you'll come to look forward to the crisp, clean, and refreshing tastes and textures of these cleansing foods as counterpoints to heavy, cloying meals of more sumptuous fare.

One of the best recovery tips is the "move right along please" approach. Your good eating will have promoted efficient function in all your organs, both of digestion and elimination, and that means particularly your bowel. Poor eating, even a single bad meal, can upset the regular and efficient working of your bowel. It can slow down, seize right up, or move like a waterfall being chased by the river. You can help your system back to normal good function and stop it from accumulating any ill effects after a bad meal by gently helping the by-products of a poor meal to pass on through.

So, as a matter of routine after any occasion of poor eating, have a light breakfast of stewed fruits with flaxseed or oat bran or yogurt. Please note this is not an exhortation to purge yourself with large quantities of laxative foods. It's a method of carefully helping your system return to good function.

Just to keep things in perspective, what's important is enjoying *both* the meal and the occasion of eating it. These techniques for recovering good order in your body should enable you to sit down happily to any meal—no matter how badly combined or unsuitable it is—and know you can get back on track and keep improving your health and figure.

FRENCH FRIES AND ALL THAT

For many people, life wouldn't be the same without hot, crispy, golden french fries—and I promised to tell you how you could eat them without any health penalty.

French fries are carbohydrate, so they mustn't be combined with proteins, which includes steak, eggs, and fish. But fries *can* be combined with other carbohydrates and Mix With Any foods. So if you want french fries, they make a wonderful meal with a huge mixed salad; or you could eat a chip butty (if you haven't been educated in the ways of the world correctly, that's a British invention, a french fries sandwich, usually with a lot of butter on the bread with ketchup or salt and vinegar as optional extras, depending on taste).

If overweight is a problem you want to solve, you might want to forgo these delights until you have your size and shape under better control. But don't despair of ever eating fries again. You *can* make an occasional day a very special Fries BFD (Best Food Day)—but only very occasionally, perhaps once every three weeks or so.

MOVING WELL AND FEELING GOOD

When embracing healthy habits in an everyday lifestyle, the one thing most people don't even want to think about is the E word—exercise.

Some people love it, others detest it, most know it would be good for them, many would like to do it more often, but the majority just can't get it together. The "don't-like-it-but-I-know-I-should-and-wish-I-could" perception gives us a clue as to how you can make exercise a part of your good life.

First of all, let's stop talking about exercise. The word is permeated with connotations of panting, sweating, straining *effort*. It's a misleading image for such a variety and range of activities; let's talk instead about *movement*.

To appreciate how easy it can be for you to use movement to improve your quality of life, you have to understand as completely as possible the role it is already playing.

Movement is made possible by your muscles. The muscles you have are essential parts of your body, just like any other part, and they're there so you can move about. When you move about, your muscles help your body work more effectively. They squeeze, pump, massage, and stimulate your organs, glands, and fluids. They help your digestion, elimination, breathing, and every process in your body.

The more you move, the better it is for your body. The better your body works, the better it is for your muscles. That's the quid pro quo of the self-sustaining ecosystem you are.

- Your movement is therefore intricately linked to your health.

The amount and type of movements you make regularly defines how your muscles develop. Your weight and shape rely on the muscles you develop and the fats and fluids that surround them. The composition of the fats and fluids around your muscles depends, to a large degree, on the amount and type of movement you regularly do.

- Your appearance, therefore, is intricately linked with your movement.

Your self-image, mental attitudes, thoughts, and feelings impose characteristic limitations on your muscle tone, your posture, and your movements. In turn, how you characteristically sit, stand, and move around reinforces your self-image, mental attitude, thoughts, and feelings.

- Your movement is intrinsic to how you feel about and see yourself.

How others perceive you is largely influenced by your body language—how you sit, stand, and move about. Whether you do so with poise, grace, and presence, and what kind of attitude you present.

• So your movement is intricately linked to the way others see you.

Nature is frugal. It does not encourage energy to be expended unnecessarily. Nature impels you, as it does all living things, to move only to the extent that it is essential for you to do so.

You are compelled to use energy in movement to the extent that it enables you to fulfill your basic needs. Stay out of trouble, get sustenance, find shelter, and locate a partner. I call this basic subsistence movement.

You, however, are not a simple animal by any stretch of the imagination. For you, it's also essential to sustain our self-image. Since movement is one way to do that, you'll be compelled to move as much as and in whatever ways will support your inner self.

In other words, how you instinctively choose to use your body in movement is an indicator as to the nature and content of your self-image. You won't, for instance, want to take part in activities and sports that don't feel as if they are "you" or how you want to be seen.

Some people are very physical and active. They indulge in fast, hard, and active sports and exercise. They may be involved in clubs and teams, or they may enjoy more solitary activities. They compete and test themselves against other people or the elements. They are validated in their view of themselves by their movements, and are helped in maintaining their perception by the adrenal and neurochemical charges they get from their activities.

Other people are physically less active. They choose enterprises involving little exercise from which to gain confirmation of their self-image. Some people don't exercise at all because that's the way they express their inner self and that's how it is best reinforced. Even when reason states they should move more, and they are wracked with regrets that they do not, they will still prevaricate and be motivated toward inactivity.

If those with an instinctive motivation to inactivity try to engage in much exercise, they rapidly feel emotionally uncomfortable and motivated to stop. They also run a greater risk than most of suffering physical harm. The very fact that they have not been inclined to move very much for a long time means they are much less capable of sustained exercise and can be easily injured.

Here, then, is an explanation which accounts for the variety of different attitudes and levels of desire involved in exercise. There is a constant trade-off between nature's basic need to conserve energy by motivating only subsistence movement and its more sophisticated role in complex human beings for self-image–driven movement. The contradictions inherent in this situation can lead to compulsive and excessive exercising on the one hand, or underactivity and guilt from unrealized good intentions on the other.

Somewhere on the spectrum between complete inactivity and frenetic exercise is You—with all your personal preconceptions about exercise—preferring to move just as much as you need in order to fulfill *your* basic needs and to express what's in *your* inner self-image. The question to be answered now is: How can you successfully include movement in your life so it helps your health and weight control?

What you do must be compatible with your self-image and present needs. It must also be regular and additional to what you are already doing, so it maintains the momentum for improvement you've already established with your Strategies.

My assumption here has to be that you are fairly inactive and don't exercise much. If you are very active and still need to improve your health or weight control, you have to consider one of two possibilities. One, the kind of activity you are doing might be unsuitable for what you want to achieve. It may even be part of the problem. Or two, your health and weight problem might be almost entirely food or mind-set associated, and your solution will be found there, not in extra exercise.

For the majority who engage in too little regular exercise, there are three things you can do to successfully include appropriate regular extra movement in your daily life.

First, take the time to find an activity you will enjoy doing. The fantastic thing about the world in which we live is the sheer variety of recreational options available to us. Use your imagination. Be creative and don't be constrained by what you think is usually meant by proper "exercise." For example, if you are completely at a loss, and can't think of any organized or formal sporting activity or exercise you'd like, just do more of what you do every day or choose a variety of activities which will add up, on average, to 10 percent more movement each day (see page 163 for the 10 Percent Rule).

Here are a few of the simplest activities you can use. Walking, golf, swimming, cycling, yoga, tai chi, making love, and cleaning and polishing. Yes! Floor polishing, car polishing, and window cleaning are all good exercise and have the added benefit of the sense of satisfaction that comes from an activity with an admirable end result.

Next, sow some seeds in your mind. Use affirmations, visualization, and positive inner dialogue to establish the idea that your chosen activity is enjoyable, beneficial, and en route to your goals.

Finally, for a reasonable period, say a month, undertake a methodical program during which you establish the extra activity into your routine. Your aim—and it may take a few weeks—is to attain a level of daily regular movement and activity that:

- Makes you feel good and as if you are getting better all the time
- Enables you to accept the belief you are gaining the body shape you will be happy with
- Keeps you as healthy as you want to be

One final point. Experiments have shown that visualizing yourself doing exercises actually improves muscle quality and performance. I believe dreaming about exercise and movement has a similar effect. So the apparently vicarious occupation of watching sports could actually be of some benefit if you really allow yourself to get into the experience.

WEAR YOURSELF OUT

Have you ever thought that your clothes could improve your health and weight control? In fact, not just your clothes, but your hair and general grooming as well? Does that seem strange to you?

Think about why there is a fashion industry at all and about how clothes, hair styling, makeup, and grooming products are marketed. You'll realize that they're aimed at your self-image. The implication is that self-image is something that can be expressed, created, recreated, exploited, and manipulated to make you happy. The idea is correct, but the methods need working on.

The industries of self-image enhancement can provide you with a benefit that you might not expect, but only if you use them in the most positive ways. Let's look more closely at yet another fascinating element of self-care—and one I hope you'll enjoy.

You can have little doubt by now that the game of health and weight control are won or lost in your mind.

Your body reinforces how you see yourself—moment by moment—with every movement, every pose, posture, and facial expression. Your poise, grace, and physical presence—or lack of them—support the reality of your inner self-model.

And of course, how you see yourself constitutes your self-image, which is at the core of the process from which your health and weight and everything about you evolves.

Just as you can consciously develop your muscles and modify your posture to give yourself better messages that will ultimately improve your self-image—and all it gives rise to—so you can use your clothes, hair style, and makeup to do the same.

You choose your clothes, hair style, and makeup for reasons. Maybe to express how you see yourself, maybe to express how you want to be seen, possibly to accentuate some aspect of your personality in particular circumstances. You might have an outdoor face and an indoor one; you could have outdoor clothes to be seen in and indoor clothes to feel relaxed in; you dress to be as you think appropriate.

By considering what you usually wear and how you present yourself, you can make sure the messages you are giving to your inner self are ones that support the you that will be healthy, happy, slim, and contented.

It's just another tactic in the mind game, one to help you maintain your momentum for improvement. By being conscious of the subtle signals you are giving to your self-image, and making sure the messages are suitable ones, every part of you will benefit.

Earlier on, you were introduced to the technique of visualization. You were encouraged to create an inner image of how you would like to be. You were asked to imagine a new self-image that you could aspire to and that your body/mind process could create and organize around. Your imagined self was to be complete with beliefs about yourself, thoughts, feelings, attitudes, posture, gestures, and movements that expressed the most healthy, happy, and contented person you could conceive of becoming.

You can also dress and groom yourself to be that way. You can bring that image more alive in your mind by taking the image from your mind's eye and actually dressing as if you were already that way.

Let me stress here, I'm not suggesting you present a mask or representation of how you think you ought to be, but that you present yourself as you are at this moment becoming. There is a huge difference.

People already dress to present masks and images they think will help them at work, or to attract a partner, or encourage friendship or attention. What they present, knowingly or not, is a false image—or at best, only a part of a self-image. I'm suggesting you have a more appropriate agenda for how you dress and groom yourself. Try to represent only what you aspire to—good health and good shape—and that you dress to represent that aspiration.

Be creative. Use color, texture, and form. Consider whether tight or loose clothing expresses how you'd like to be. Don't just think about your outer wear—apply the same ideas to your underwear, shoes, hair, makeup, and jewelry.

I recall one client whose bra was a monument to the concept that "fashion is more important than function." So long had she worn foundation wear featuring narrow lacy straps (on an item otherwise designed for her very large bust) that the straps had virtually embedded themselves in her shoulders. She actually had a groove on each shoulder into which the straps slotted every time she put on her bra!

With some misgivings and not a little hint of concern about the fashion statement she was making, the lady changed, on my insistence, to a bra with wider straps. The result, within a short time, was relief from severe neck pain and loss of sensation in her fingers that were the reasons she had called me. She found she could walk straighter, with her shoulders back, and within a short time her entire demeanor changed to become more relaxed and happy in general. I'll let *you* imagine the benefits of changing from overtight underpants.

Ask yourself the question "If I was as happy, healthy, and content as I could be, how would I look?" Now go and dress yourself to look that way.

Use your grooming as a powerful affirmation of your continuing self-care and a way of sustaining your enthusiasm. Make what you wear and how you wear it a demonstration of your intention to act for your best health and shape.

Clothing and hair are sensory realities of which we can seem unaware. But they are constantly with us and are consistent sources of good or bad messages to your self-image, without your realizing it, every time you move or look at yourself in a mirror.

One last thing—can I *please* beg you not to wear backless, slip-on shoes! They can't keep your feet warm properly, they don't look nice, and above all you can't walk well when you're sluffing around in them. When my clients complain about aching feet and legs, the first item I check is their footwear—and I usually find mules, slippers, flip-flops, or whatever else you may care to call them. If nothing else, wear shoes in which you can walk well, with confident strides in elegance and grace—or wear no shoes at all.

REAL RICHNESS

I know who I was when I woke up this morning, but I think I must have changed several times since then.
—Lewis Carroll, *Alice's Adventures in Wonderland*

Change is inevitable, and whether you wish it or not you will be a different person tomorrow than you are today. You'll be changed at the most fundamental level by the death and regeneration of cells in every part of your body except your brain. There cells will die but not be replaced.

Your mind will be changed too. New information will give you a different perspective on the world, a new reality. New experiences will give you a new view of yourself, a new self-image. The changes may be so slight you do not notice them, or so substantial you know immediately that something is different.

However great or small the changes, your life will be different because of them. Cellular changes mean the body that lives through each day is a different body the next, and then a different one again as the process of change continues. Differences that arise in your mind eventually bring about profound changes to your body as well.

Your changing reality and altering self-image means your frame of reference is constantly shifting, and with each change to the way you see yourself and the world comes a change to the choices and decisions you make. Change is the way of Life. It is continuous and inexorable.

Your changing will be largely spontaneous and unplanned, and the outcome will be uncertain *unless* you become aware of what is happening and involve yourself in the process. Awareness and involvement require two things from you. First, a conscious mental process in which *you plan* the nature of the change you want to make, as opposed to accepting that which will occur without your participation. Second, some *action* on your part to achieve the changes you prefer.

The *Love Food . . . Lose Weight* diet sets in motion a body/mind process that acknowledges and utilizes this process of change to improve your health and weight control.

Awareness, involvement, choice, and action are inherent in every strategy and technique for self-improvement you have learned. The actual degree of those improvements and the rate at which they will occur is impossible to predict, but they *will* come about. And there is something more.

Your new self-image—inevitable if you follow basic guidelines—will generate changes of a more subtle nature. You will find yourself making different choices in many areas of your life; you will discover yourself being drawn to new and different experiences. Because your intention is for positive change and because the methods employed are life-enhancing and enabling, the outcomes will be positive and empowering. In short, your life will spontaneously get better in ways you cannot yet imagine.

But you *can* engage yourself more closely in this aspect of your transformation. Here are two ways you might want to consider.

First, in my experience, people improve much more rapidly and beneficially when they are involved in some kind of constructive pastime. It might be a career, but it can just as easily be a hobby, a sport, or a charity. The essential point is that it is *meaningful* to you—that you get satisfaction from what you do. What you do must validate the best you see in yourself. Equally important is that you don't choose to do anything you feel is not worthy of you. This is golden advice.

A significant element of the body/mind process is that it has direction and purpose. Using your time in a way that feels good and valuable for you provides that direction and purpose. You'll experience a definite sense of well-being when you engage yourself in such endeavor.

The other way to help yourself is to use a simple mind process. There is a question you can put to yourself which will take you to the core of what is most supportive for you. If, for instance, you realize you are feeling or doing something you would prefer not to, you can ask this question of yourself. If you are faced with a choice or decision in any area of your life, you can ask yourself this in relation to any of the options:

"What must I believe about myself for this to be happening for me?"

Take a moment to ask yourself that question when you realize you are doing or feeling something you prefer not to, and you will discover the belief which is at the core of your uncertainty Use it when you are faced with a decision, and you will know what you must believe to make an option work for you.

You know that beliefs are learned. New beliefs can be learned and old ones superseded. Your life quest is to acquire the best beliefs you can, the beliefs that will underpin your best health, your best weight, and your most empowering and joyful lifestyle. And on that journey *Love Food . . . Lose Weight* will be your faithful guide.

Delicious Meals for Perfect Health

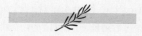

This chapter brings all you've learned so far to where it matters most—the food on your plate. It's here you'll find just how spectacular, how revolutionary, and how exciting the *Love Food . . . Lose Weight* way of food combining is!

The recipes which follow adhere strictly to the basic food-combining rule: Eat your protein and carbohydrate foods separately, so they will not be in your stomach at the same time. That's just where the fun starts, though, because I've designed these recipes to show how you can make food combining quick, simple, and utterly delicious. These recipes are the ones you'll need if you're going to follow the Daily Menu Options from the Master Plan. Whether you're following the Master Plan, making up your own menus, or are just at a loss for a meal idea, you can turn to this chapter with complete confidence.

One of the most common incentives for failing at any diet is if the food you have to eat makes you feel deprived. A wonderful way of overcoming such built-in discouragement is to make your healthy meals more exciting and flavorful than the unhealthy meals you're used to.

The *Love Food . . . Lose Weight* recipes are delicious in their own right, but you'll notice I often use small amounts of especially tasty foods to create stunning flavor combinations—with occasional taste sensations—that will pepper your meals with mouthfuls of sheer pleasure. Please do try these suggestions, and explore the shelves of your nearest deli or ethnic grocer until you build a collection of taste embellishments—you'll never look back.

TASTE SENSATIONS

- *Oils:* Sesame, walnut, and hazelnut oils will lift a salad, plate of crudités, or a simple baked potato—just sprinkle half a dozen drops over all.
- *Sauces:* I remember the famous travel writer Paul Theroux once said that he always took a bottle of Tabasco with him to whatever country he visited because it made *anything* edible—and two or three drops of the infamous Tabasco sauce could be all you need to transform "good" into "wonderful." Also, consider trying horseradish, mustard, and mint sauces. Chinese and other Asian grocery stores stock their own form of ginger paste—a teaspoon on the side of your plate provides a convenient dip for crudités.
- *Condiments:* Good old salt and pepper . . . But have you tried the Chinese five spice or spices for couscous mixtures which you can buy at a delicatessen or good supermarket? A pinch of either of these will give surprise and zest to countless meals. Now, take a closer look at all those spices you have been walking past all these years: cayenne, paprika, anise or fennel seed, nutmeg, cinnamon and ginger, both dried and freshly grated.
- *Herbs:* fresh or dried, blended with oil into purées or added to sauces and soups bring taste sensations which can add completely new dimensions of flavor to your meals. And many have a beneficial effect on your health as well.

Another way of lifting yourself and your food out of the diet doldrums is to place extra emphasis on the presentation of your meal. Whether it's just for yourself or for others as well, food that looks great on the plate seems to taste better and satisfy more. These are only initial suggestions, though, to alert you to the possibilities for expressing your personal style when you cook the *Love Food . . . Lose Weight* way.

PRESENTATION TIPS

Let me give you just a quick-fix collection of presentation tips to get you started. Most people don't need much encouragement to make great presentations of food for their loved ones, friends, and venerated others. I suggest you also try to treat *yourself* to superlative presentations of your own meals, even when you eat alone. It really brings quality to your meal. Care in presentation means showing care—care for yourself, too.

First, when choosing the plate or bowl in which to serve your meal, consider three things.

1. Make sure the dish is generous in size so that the food can be moved around a little while you eat. I know one famous chain of restaurants which serves their meals in such skimpy dishes that even the most fastidious eater spills much of the first few bites all over the table.
2. Try to choose a dish whose color and/or pattern will enhance the food rather than make it appear repellent.
3. Find a dish that suits the food. You wouldn't usually serve soup on a saucer, would you? Think of whether the food is splashy, drippy, needs slicing or some form of dismantling during the meal—then pick your dish to suit.

Next is what I term the Pause Factor. This is the response that happens when you present a meal effectively. When the plate looks more than just right, when it looks fantastic, delectable, tantalizing, then the person who receives it will pause and enjoy it just as it is for a few precious seconds before digging in. There are five points to check out before you can count on that response.

1. Texture must be obvious in the meal you serve. In fact, three different textures in the food items are about the minimum you should aim for before you can expect the response. That's why, in any recipe you read, some ingredients will be described by their texture: finely chopped, crushed, sliced julienne, roughly torn, and so on. On your plate, count the

textures and try to arrange them in a dramatic and pleasing way.

2. Color has an almost instantaneous effect, and if it's not right, the whole meal is in question. Aim for soft backgrounds, deep, rich tones in places and one or two sharp color contrasts to tie the whole thing together. Use the plate or a serving of grains, purée, or sauce as the soft background, the oranges and deep yellows of carrots and pumpkins and the luscious dark greens of broccoli and spinach, for instance, as the rich tones. Your garnish or a dollop of sauce can be the sharp contrast.

3. Pattern or picture is important, as emphasized so well in the Nouvelle Cuisine style made popular in recent years. But even if you have no heart for that style of presentation, there is a definite feeling which happens when a meal has been carefully placed on the plate. Experiment.

4. Expectation of what the meal will include is sometimes involved in the pause response. If you expect one steak—be it beef or bean—and three veg, then you anticipate a certain look to the plate. And it takes a lot to get a good response if that look doesn't happen! Whether or not you know what your meal consists of, you will still have expectations. For instance, if there is a dry part, you'll expect a wet part to go with it. If there is hard stuff, you'll expect soft stuff, too. If there is something to be soaked in or dipped into, you'll expect something to do the soaking up or dipping. Try to meet expectations, but do it creatively and with as much fun and flair as you can muster.

5. Garnish is that little bit of something or other that may be thrown away at the end of the meal, but at the moment of presentation it does its bit. Garnish is the final touch for color, texture, and placement or proportion of the meal on the plate. It may also be a taste sensation and it can, if you let yourself, have a bit of quirky or poetical expression.

Finally, presentation creates the pause response when everything else is just right, too. For some that means the place mat being properly aligned, for others the right music in the background. Please take the opportunity each mealtime to explore the total environment of your meal so that you can elevate it to a peaceful, pleasurable occasion.

Some years ago I spent many months studying the Japanese tea ceremony. Every element of these beautiful ceremonies—there are actually several forms—is intended to establish a place and period of serenity and beauty. From the flower arrangement and calligraphy poem, the choice of tea bowl and water jar, to the sweet foods arranged on their special lacquered tray and even the arrangement of the powdered green tea within its lacquered caddy right through to every movement and gesture, each is intended to enhance the occasion for the honored guest who has been invited to experience tea. You can show the intention behind your meal to whoever eats with you, even if it's simply yourself, by how you present your food.

In addition to creating meals which are quick, easy, and versatile, I want these recipes to stimulate your imagination about well-combined food so you'll be able to create your own recipes and develop your own style and flair for the *Love Food . . . Lose Weight* way of cooking and eating. But any meal, no matter how well designed, is only as good as its ingredients. I urge you to purchase the best ingredients you can and to gradually restock your cupboard with even the "basics" boasting real quality. Treat yourself as well as you want to be treated. Here are a few of my shopping suggestions.

SHOPPING TIPS

I use good-quality, cold-pressed virgin olive oil, preferably Italian, though Greek is also excellent. Then, as I indicate in the recipes, I keep a collection of unusual nut oils on hand to add Taste Sensations to salads, crudités, and even pasta.

It is easy to get high-quality vinegars these days, and even quite exotic ones are not so difficult to find. I use both red and white wine vinegars, apple cider vinegar (organic if possible), raspberry vinegar, balsamic vinegar, and then anything else I come across gets a "special purchase" order! I have treasured bottles of tarragon vinegar, lemon vinegar, and even a basil vinegar.

I regularly explore, with a real sense of adventure, the shelves of

Chinese and other Asian groceries to see if I can discover a new sauce or spread to tantalize my taste buds.

Fruits and vegetables are best eaten as fresh as possible.

Grains? Well, there's a whole variety to choose from. There's amaranth, quinoa, buckwheat, corn, oats, rye, spelt, rice, millet, wild rice . . . You see? Move over, wheat!

Shopping should become a pleasurable part of your food experience. It becomes enjoyable when you use quality, variety, and a sense of adventure as guides to your shopping list.

Now let's look at some of the dishes you will prepare frequently.

Salads

Salads are used as appetizers, main courses, and desserts throughout the Master Plan and at all times are open to your personal interpretation and preferences. It would be unreasonable, for instance, to specify exactly what salad greens, herbs, or other Mix With Any foods you should include every time a salad is indicated. Instead, when salad appears as an Option, I'll give you some guidelines about what I have in mind, then *you* can choose the actual items you want. A list of example ingredients to choose from is shown below.

If the salad requires some special ingredient or a specific dressing, I'll let you know the details. Otherwise simply refer to this list of Mix With Any salad ingredients; they can be used at any time, in the same meal with either carbohydrate or protein foods.

Salad Ingredients Food Category = Mix With Any (M/A)

- Salad greens: including romaine lettuce, red lettuce, green leaf lettuce, spinach, alfalfa sprouts, napa (or Chinese) cabbage, chicory, radicchio, dandelion. Try to avoid serving just iceberg lettuce and aim for a mixture of leaves to improve the flavor, texture, and nutritional value of your salad.
- Fresh herbs of all kinds can be used too. Most common are dill, mint, coriander, parsley, and basil, but chives, tarragon, sage, and fennel are also exquisite additions which can provide the aromas and flavors you'll start to look forward to in your salads.

- Unusual additions make a welcome, sometimes seasonal change. Try thinly sliced ginger root, capers, dill pickles, green and black olives, or thinly sliced water chestnuts. Raw snow peas and small peas are pleasant surprises, and fine green beans can be plunged into boiling, slightly salted water for just three or four minutes, then quickly turned into cold water to stop them cooking and keep them fresh for your salad.
- Dress your salads with a basic vinaigrette for first and main courses, and a slightly sweeter version—a dessert vinaigrette—for dessert salads. Even when using vinaigrette, though, I prefer to add variations to the dressings that will bring a little something different to each salad. I'll make suggestions as we go along.

I prefer not to create food that tastes the same throughout, no matter how good the main flavoring may be. A salad or vegetable dish that tastes identical at each mouthful because it's dressed or flavored uniformly soon gets boring. Instead, I'll make suggestions for adding taste sensations on top of excellent dressings that will make your good food even more exciting and enjoyable.

Basic Vinaigrette
Food category = Mix With Any (M/A)

INGREDIENTS

*1 tablespoon white wine vinegar
or cider vinegar*
4 tablespoons olive oil
1 teaspoon smooth Dijon mustard
½ teaspoon fine sea salt

*½ teaspoon clear honey or soft
brown sugar, optional*
*2 cloves garlic, finely crushed,
optional*
5 drops Tabasco sauce, optional

METHOD

Basic proportions are 1 part of vinegar to 4 parts of oil. The recipe for a standard portion which can be multiplied according to need:

Measure the ingredients into a large screw-top jar. Screw down the top of the jar and shake vigorously until the ingredients blend into a smooth dressing. Alternatively, mix all the ingredients except the oil in a large bowl, then whisk in the oil, a little at a time, to produce the same end result.

VARIATIONS

Add finely chopped fresh herbs of your choice. For instance, basil goes well with a tomato salad; dill with a cucumber salad; tarragon with a salad containing artichokes or mushrooms; a salad with lots of onion or olives benefits from finely chopped fennel leaf.

Replace a proportion of the olive oil with a delicious nut oil such as walnut or hazelnut, now widely available in supermarkets and health food shops.

Dessert Vinaigrette

Food category = Mix With Any (M/A)

INGREDIENTS

1 tablespoon white wine vinegar
or cider vinegar
4 tablespoons olive oil
1 teaspoon smooth Dijon
mustard

½ teaspoon fine sea salt
1 teaspoon clear honey or soft
brown sugar, optional
1 clove garlic, finely crushed,
optional

METHOD

Basic proportions are 1 part of vinegar to 4 parts of oil or a standard portion which can be multiplied according to need:

Measure the ingredients into a large screw-top jar. Screw down the top of the jar and shake vigorously until the ingredients blend into a smooth dressing. Alternatively, mix all the ingredients except the oil in a large bowl, then whisk in the oil, a little at a time, to produce the same end result.

VARIATIONS

Delightful flavor surprises can be created by using a fruit vinegar such as lemon or raspberry, or a rose petal vinegar. Now's your chance to browse through your local delicatessen.

Crudités

Food category = Mix With Any (M/A)

Crudités are used quite often in the Master Plan as a starter course. It helps to have some ideas from which to choose your selection of crudités, so here's a list to get your imagination working.

These are just a few of the vegetables you can enjoy in their raw state: celery sticks, carrot sticks, slices or separate leaves of chicory, florets of cauliflower or broccoli, slices of red, green, or yellow peppers, whole snow peas, slices of sweet onion, slices of zucchini, thin slices of fennel, slices or leaves of lettuce, radicchio, turnip sticks, red radish, sliced kohlrabi, cucumber.

Prepare your crudités: clean and trim your chosen vegetables well and refresh them in clean, cold water, then cut them into pieces suitable for dipping or spreading with the accompaniment you've selected.

If weight control is important to you, crudités are a filling first course, with plenty of fiber, few calories, and no fat. They are the ideal way to start a meal and take the edge off a hunger which might otherwise lead you to overeat from another course with a bigger weight gain penalty.

Vegetable Stock

In the *Love Food . . . Lose Weight* recipes, vegetable stock is used extensively for poaching and as the basis for soups and sauces. Using vegetable stock is a good way of recovering nutrients lost when vegetables are cooked, simply by including their cooking liquor in the stock. It also means that just Mix With Any foods are being used, which removes any rotation and combining problems that can arise from using protein-based stocks such as fish, beef, or chicken.

Some recipes occasionally benefit from a protein-based stock, and when within the food-combining rules, it is OK to use one even when it results in mixing different proteins in a meal. For example, you might want to use chicken stock for a soup before a main course which includes fish.

For the moment, though, I recommend you keep your meals simple whenever you can, and avoid mixing too many proteins together. For that reason the *Love Food . . . Lose Weight* recipes recommend vegetable stock.

The best thing to do is to regularly make up fresh amounts of your Basic Vegetable Stock and keep some available all the time. Stock from the recipe which follows can be kept in an airtight container for up to three days in your refrigerator and up to three months in your freezer.

To freeze your home-made stock:

Line a one- or two-cup bowl or straight-sided jar with a large freezer bag. Leave the stock to cool to room temperature, then pour a premeasured amount of stock into the bag before putting it, bowl and all, into the freezer. When the stock is frozen you can seal the bag, remove it from the bowl or jug, and keep it frozen for up to three months, or until you need it. Simply remove one or two bags from the freezer and turn their contents into the pot.

Commercial vegetable stock cubes can be used, but they vary considerably in quality. Many contain additives (such as monosodium glutamate), colorings, and flavorings which are not needed in your food. Others have such a high salt content and hardly any other flavor that they do little to enhance your food and frequently spoil it with the excess salt.

I do use them occasionally, however; I suggest you experiment until you find one you can get from your health food shop or supermarket. Then keep a package available as a backup, in case you need stock very quickly, or to strengthen the flavor of your own stock. Vegetable stock, canned or from the freezer section of most supermarkets, is also a good option if you don't have your own available.

Anyway, here's the recipe for Basic Vegetable Stock. It's really easy and well worth taking a little time to make it.

Basic Vegetable Stock

Food category = Mix With Any (M/A)

INGREDIENTS

2 tablespoons olive oil

3–4 medium carrots, washed,
   trimmed, and coarsely chopped

2 medium onions, chopped

2 bay leaves

small bunch fresh thyme

4 stalks celery, washed and
   coarsely chopped

2 leeks, washed, trimmed, and
   coarsely chopped

6 whole black peppercorns

6¼ cups cold water

METHOD

Place a large saucepan or stock pot over a low heat, warm the oil, then add the vegetables, herbs, and peppercorns. Cook, stirring occasionally, until the onions are clear and the vegetables are softening, about 5–10 minutes.

Add the water and bring to a simmer. Simmer uncovered for 30–40 minutes until the stock is reduced by about one-third.

Strain stock through a fine sieve. Use immediately or store for later use.

VARIATIONS

Changes to this Basic Stock can be made during preparation or at the time the stock is used by adding garlic, other herbs, or spices suitable for the main dish with which you want to use it. Salt and pepper seasoning should only be added to the final recipe.

A small beet, washed and trimmed, may be added to the stock to give it a beautiful ruby color and earthy flavor.

Desserts

My assumption is that you want to control your weight and improve your health, and frequent indulgence in big, sticky, high-fat, high-sugar, and high-calorie desserts is not compatible with that aim. I've therefore suggested desserts which will give you refreshing or exciting tastes with which to end your meal.

If you're a cake person, and have to have a real, blow-out-your cheeks dessert, I suggest you replace one meal, very occasionally, with just that. Start with a light salad and make your main course a wonderful dessert from just what the doctor didn't order—but make sure the ingredients are properly combined.

I've already mentioned that one of my favorite desserts is a glass of sweet wine with one or two high-quality chocolates. Try it—it's great, and perfectly self-indulgent.

THE MASTER PLAN RECIPE COLLECTION

To make it easy for you to follow the meals recommended in the Master Plan, the recipes below are arranged in the same sequence as they appear in the Daily Menu Options in chapter 3. Please use the general tips for Salads, Crudités, and Desserts, above. Here now are your *Love Food . . . Lose Weight* recipes.

Recipes

Day 1 Option A

Mushroom Soup

Food category = Mix With Any (M/A)

SERVES **4**

INGREDIENTS

2–3 tablespoons olive oil
1 large onion, finely diced
1 pound white or brown
   mushrooms cleaned
   and sliced (or substitute
   one quarter with shiitake and/
   or oyster mushrooms). Keep
   2 small mushrooms whole
   and to one side for garnish
pinch freshly grated nutmeg
2 tablespoons dry sherry
   (or white wine)

2½ cups Basic Vegetable Stock (see
   page 194)
1 small clove garlic, chopped,
   optional
sea salt and freshly ground black
   pepper, to taste
lemon juice, to taste
2 tablespoons light cream, to taste
2 tablespoons finely chopped fresh
   chives, optional

METHOD

Heat 2 tablespoons of the oil in a large saucepan over low heat. Sauté the chopped onion, stirring occasionally, until it is clear and tender, but not browned.

Add the sliced mushrooms, nutmeg, sherry or wine, two-thirds of the vegetable stock, and the garlic, if used. Season lightly with salt and black pepper (do not add salt if using stock cubes). Bring to simmer, stirring occasionally, and simmer covered for 15 minutes.

Meanwhile, slice the 2 small mushrooms kept for garnish, and fry them quickly in a little hot oil until just browned and crisp. Set them aside on a paper towel to drain. If a chunky soup is preferred, remove 2 or 3 tablespoons of sliced mushrooms from the soup to a bowl and keep them to one side. Purée the soup in a blender or food processor until smooth. If a very smooth soup is required, pass it through a fine sieve.

Return the soup to the pan and add the mushroom slices removed prior to blending. Keep the soup warm but not simmering while you adjust the consistency and flavor by adding the remaining stock, lemon juice to taste, light cream and further seasoning of salt and freshly ground black pepper. Serve in warm bowls topped with the crisp mushroom slices and finely chopped chives, if used.

TIP
A lighter soup can be made by replacing the cream with up to 1 cup of skim milk. However, this will make it a protein soup, suitable only for use in meals containing proteins and no carbohydrates.

VARIATION
Try topping with a spoonful of finely chopped mushrooms sautéed until soft with chopped parsley, in place of the fried mushroom slices.

Couscous and Mixed Vegetables with Piquant Sauce

Food category = Carbohydrate (C)

SERVES 4

INGREDIENTS

2 tablespoons olive oil

1 medium onion, finely chopped

½ teaspoon ground paprika

½ teaspoon ground turmeric

½ teaspoon ground cumin

½ teaspoon ground ginger

½ teaspoon ground cinnamon

2½ cups Basic Vegetable Stock (see page 194)

1 cup small onions, quartered

1 cup carrots, diced (¾ inch wide)

1 cup turnips, diced (¾ inch wide)

1 cup cauliflower, as florets

1 cup sliced (¾ inch wide) leeks

4½ cups cold water

1 cup zucchini, sliced

12 ounces quick-cook couscous

2 tablespoons finely chopped fresh cilantro

3 ripe medium tomatoes, peeled, seeded, and chopped

1 teaspoon chopped fresh chili pepper, seeded

1 small clove garlic, optional

sea salt and freshly ground black pepper, to taste

Tabasco sauce, to taste

You'll also need a vegetable steamer for this recipe. A fan steamer placed in the bottom of a large saucepan will work if you don't have the more sophisticated stacking kind.

METHOD

Heat the oil in a large saucepan suitable for steaming. Sauté the finely chopped onion and all the ground spices over low heat, stirring occasionally until the onion is soft but not browning, about 5–10 minutes.

Add some of the stock to the sauté—enough liquid to steam the vegetables, but not to touch them if they are in a fan steamer over the stock. To a depth of ½–¾ inch is usually fine. Bring the stock to a simmer with the steamer and lid in place.

Put the quartered onions, carrots, and turnips in the steamer and steam, covered, for 10 minutes. Add a little more stock, then add the cauliflower florets. Cover and steam for 2 minutes. Add a little more stock, then add the leeks, cover and steam for 2 minutes. Add a little more stock, then add the zucchini, cover and steam for up to 5 minutes until all the vegetables are cooked but still firm. About 20 minutes in total.

Meanwhile, boil 3½ cups of water in a kettle. Measure the couscous into a large bowl or saucepan and pour the boiling water over. Stir well, cover, and leave to stand.

Turn all the steamed vegetables into a large, warm serving dish and gently mix in the fresh cilantro.

Add the chopped tomatoes, chopped chili, remaining stock, and the garlic, if used, to the steaming stock and simmer rapidly for 2 minutes. Add a little water if necessary to make 2–3 cups of sauce. Adjust the sauce to taste with salt and pepper and pour it over the vegetables.

Turn the couscous into another large bowl and let each person help themselves to a plate of couscous, top it with vegetables in the piquant sauce, then add Tabasco sauce as desired.

VARIATION

Instead of steaming the vegetables they can be poached in the stock. Poach all the root vegetables together in about a cup of stock with the sauté for 10 minutes, then add the leeks and cauliflower for 5 minutes more, then add the zucchini for the remainder of 20 minutes until all the vegetables are cooked but still a little firm, adding more stock if necessary.

Remove the vegetables to the warm serving bowl and mix in the cilantro, retaining the stock in the pan.

Add the chopped tomatoes, chili, remaining stock and garlic, and continue as in the original recipe.

To quarter the small onions so the sections are about the same size as the other vegetable pieces, peel the outer skin back, leaving the root intact. Trim the skin off near the root so each onion is kept whole by the remaining root core. Then slice the onions top to bottom through the root core to make correctly sized sections of onion.

Mint Ice

Food category = Carbohydrate (C)

SERVES **4**

INGREDIENTS

⅔ cup granulated sugar
1 cup cold water
1 tablespoon honey
1 tablespoon lemon juice

1 tablespoon lime juice
⅓ cup mint liqueur
fresh mint sprigs, for garnish

METHOD

In a large, heavy-based saucepan dissolve the sugar in the water and bring to boil over moderate heat. Remove from heat and allow to cool.

Add honey, lemon and lime juices, and two-thirds of the mint liqueur, mix well until the honey is dissolved, then transfer to a large bowl or tub for freezing. Place the bowl in the freezer and freeze the mixture until partially frozen. Ice crystals should be forming around the edges of the bowl.

Remove the bowl from the freezer and beat the mixture until the ice crystals are dispersed. You can do this with a fork or more rapidly in a blender or food processor.

Return the bowl to the freezer and repeat the beating/blending twice more until the mixture is firming up evenly. Allow the Mint Ice to freeze firm.

Place the Mint Ice in the refrigerator about 30 minutes before serving time, to soften. Scoop into cold dessert dishes or robust glasses, drizzle a little of the remaining third of the mint liqueur over each, and add a sprig of mint for garnish.

Smoked Salmon Salad

Food category = Protein (P)

SERVES 4

INGREDIENTS

mixed salad greens, your
choice (e.g., romaine,
spinach, red lettuce),
washed and dried
lemon juice
nut oil, your choice (e.g.,
walnut or hazelnut)
8 ounces smoked salmon,
thinly sliced or cut into
½-inch strips

2 tablespoons capers
2 tablespoons finely chopped
fresh herb (e.g.,dill or chives)
freshly ground black pepper, to
taste
Tabasco sauce, optional

METHOD

Wash and crisp the salad greens in cold water, drain and pat or spin
dry. Coarsely tear the leaves and toss together in a large bowl. Dress
the leaves by drizzling them with a little lemon juice and nut oil to
your taste, mixing gently until all the leaves are lightly flavored.
Arrange the leaves onto each of four plates.

Arrange about 2 ounces of the sliced smoked salmon over the
leaves on each plate. Scatter a teaspoon or so of capers onto each
salad, sprinkle each with about a teaspoon of chopped fresh dill or
chives.

Grind a little black pepper on each salad and sprinkle a few drops
of Tabasco on each if desired. Serve immediately.

VARIATION

Replace 4 ounces of the smoked salmon with a small jar of large red
salmon roe. The method is the same.

Turkey Cutlets, Ribbon Vegetables, and Herb Sauce

Food category = Protein (P)

SERVES **4**

INGREDIENTS

turkey steaks or cutlets (thin slices), approximately 4–5 ounces per person

olive oil

sea salt and freshly ground black pepper, to taste

4 medium carrots, peeled and shaved into ribbons

4 medium zucchini, trimmed and shaved into ribbons

4 medium leeks, trimmed and sliced into ribbons

2½ cups Basic Vegetable Stock (see page 194)

1 bunch fresh thyme

3–4 ounces unsalted butter at room temperature

½ cup finely chopped fresh parsley

4 small sprigs thyme, for garnish

METHOD

Gently beat out the turkey steaks or cutlets between plastic wrap, to approximately half inch thick, but not so much that they begin to disintegrate. Brush the cutlets with a little olive oil and season on both sides with a little sea salt and freshly ground black pepper. Set aside between fresh plastic wrap to await cooking. Line the broiler pan with foil and oil the broiler rack with olive oil.

Heat the oven to 150°F and warm four serving plates and a large serving bowl for the vegetable ribbons.

Prepare the vegetables by cutting into ribbons (see below).

Put 1 cup of the vegetable stock and the bunch of thyme in a large saucepan or wok over medium heat and bring to a boil.

Remove the thyme and retain for further use. Add the carrot ribbons to the stock, cover, and poach for 4–5 minutes, until just beginning to soften. Lift the carrot ribbons from the stock and put them in the warm, covered serving bowl in the oven. Pour off and retain the stock. Bring 1 cup of stock to a boil with the bunch of thyme, then remove the thyme, add the leek ribbons, cover, and poach for 3–4 minutes, until soft. Lift the leek ribbons from the stock and place in the bowl with the carrots.

Meanwhile, start broiling the turkey. Arrange the turkey cutlets on the broiler rack. The cutlets will need 4–5 minutes on each side.

Replace the bunch of thyme in the stock and bring to a boil, remove the thyme, add the zucchini ribbons, cover, and poach for 2–3 minutes, until just soft. Lift the zucchini ribbons from the stock and place in the warm serving bowl.

Add the retained stock from the carrots, then measure 1 cup of cooking stock into a small saucepan and bring to a simmer with the thyme. Measure 1 cup of stock and bring it to a simmer with the thyme. Remove the thyme and whisk in up to 3 ounces of the butter, a little at a time, to make a smooth butter sauce. If it remains a little thin or you want it smoother, whisk in the remaining butter. A hand-held blender helps. Add the chopped parsley to the butter sauce, stir it well.

To serve, share the sauce between the four warm plates. Arrange a turkey cutlet on each plate and garnish each with a small sprig of thyme. Gently toss the vegetable ribbons together in the bowl and season with freshly ground black pepper. Serve.

VARIATION

The vegetables are equally enjoyable and cook just as quickly if the carrots and zucchini (not the pulp) are sliced into long julienne "noodles" instead of ribbons. The cooking method is the same as described.

HOW TO MAKE VEGETABLE RIBBONS

With a swivel-type potato peeler, shave the carrots and zucchini into ribbons—as though peeling them right down to their core. Keep the carrot ribbons separated from the zucchini. Work around the zucchini taking some green outer skin with white flesh for each ribbon. Discard the pulp from the center or use in your next batch of vegetable stock. Cut the leeks lengthwise in half, then in quarters, then each quarter into quarters again. Suddenly you have leek ribbons! Parsnips, rutabaga, turnip, cucumber, and many other vegetables may be prepared and presented in this way. The appearance is light and, if the ribbons are mixed, very colorful as well.

Tomato Salad with Dessert Vinaigrette

Food category = Mix With Any (M/A)

SERVES 4

INGREDIENTS

5–6 tablespoons Dessert
   Vinaigrette (see page 191)
2 large ripe (beef)
   tomatoes, thinly sliced
2 medium carrots, finely grated

1 small sweet (or green) onion, very
   finely chopped, optional
maple syrup, optional
ground cinnamon, optional

METHOD

Prepare the salad dressing.

Arrange the tomato slices onto four dessert plates or dishes. Top with grated carrot and chopped onion.

Dress each with about 1 tablespoon of Dessert Vinaigrette. Lightly drizzle with maple syrup and sprinkle with a pinch of cinnamon, if used. Serve.

VARIATION

A mixture of finely chopped fresh basil and celery leaves may be sprinkled over the grated carrot instead of—or as well as—the chopped onion and cinnamon.

Day 1 Option B

Spinach and Pea Soup
Food category = Mix With Any (M/A)

SERVES 4

INGREDIENTS

1 pound fresh or frozen
  leaf spinach (thawed)
2 tablespoons olive oil
1 large onion, finely chopped
pinch freshly grated nutmeg
3½ cups Basic Vegetable
  Stock (see page 194)

sea salt and freshly ground black
  pepper, to taste
6 frozen petit pois (small peas)
light cream, to taste (up to
  2 tablespoons)
whole fine chives, for garnish

METHOD

Wash, trim, and spin or shake dry the fresh spinach, if used.

Heat the oil in a large saucepan over low heat and sauté the chopped onion, stirring occasionally, until the onion is clear and tender, without browning. Add the spinach, nutmeg, and half a cup of the vegetable stock. Season lightly (if using stock cubes, do not add salt). Stir well, bring to a simmer, cover, and cook for 5 minutes.

Add the petit pois (peas), bring back to a simmer, and cook for a further 3 minutes. Meanwhile, wash 2–3 whole fine chives for each person, and set them aside on a paper towel to dry.

Purée the vegetables in a blender or food processor with all but 1 cup of the remaining stock. If a very smooth soup is required, pass it through a fine sieve. Return the soup to the pan and keep it warm but not simmering while you adjust the consistency and flavor to your taste by adding the remaining stock, light cream, and further seasoning if required. Serve in warm bowls garnished with chives.

VARIATION

A lighter soup can be made by replacing the cream with up to 1¼ cups of skim milk, but this will make it a protein soup, suitable only for use in meals containing proteins and no carbohydrates.

Salmon with Vegetables and Spinach Sauce

Food category = Protein (P)

SERVES **4**

INGREDIENTS

4 trimmed salmon steaks or
  skinned tail fillets, about
  4–5 ounces per person
1 tablespoon finely chopped
  shallot
balsamic vinegar
olive oil
1 heaped teaspoon
  fresh dill, finely chopped
  or ½ teaspoon dried)

sea salt and freshly ground
  black pepper, to taste
2½ cups Basic Vegetable Stock
  (see page 194)
4 medium carrots, peeled, trimmed,
  and roughly diced
3 ounces unsalted butter
8 medium zucchini, sliced
  lengthwise into 6–8 strips
4 small sprigs watercress, for
  garnish

FOR THE SAUCE

1¼ cups Basic Vegetable
  Stock (see page 194)
1 tablespoon lemon juice

3 good-sized bunches
  spinach, chopped
light cream, to taste

METHOD

Preheat the oven to 350°F, and preheat a baking sheet and two serving dishes also. Prepare your packages (see below). Place your packages on the hot baking sheet and bake for 20 minutes.

To prepare the carrots, bring 1¼ cups of vegetable stock to a boil in a large saucepan. Add the chopped carrots and simmer until soft, about 15 minutes. Lift the carrots from the stock and purée them with 2 ounces butter in a food processor or by pushing them through a fine sieve. Add salt and pepper to taste and adjust the consistency to a firm purée, adding stock if necessary. Turn into a hot serving dish and set aside in a warm place.

To prepare the zucchini, heat a tablespoon of olive oil and a good knob of butter in a heavy-based frying pan. Sauté the zucchini slices until just browning and soft. Drain on paper towels and arrange on a hot serving dish.

When the fish packages are cooked, remove them from the oven and put the serving plates in to warm. Cut one end of each package and drain off the liquid through a strainer into a bowl.

Make the sauce by bringing 1¼ cups of vegetable stock to a boil in a saucepan with the lemon juice, fish juices, and spinach. Simmer for 2 minutes. Blend in a food processor or with a hand blender to make a thick smooth sauce, adjust the flavor with salt, pepper, and light cream to taste.

Serve the fish on each of four warm plates. Add scoops of carrot purée, a portion of zucchini, and a generous topping of spinach sauce over all. Serve immediately.

HOW TO PREPARE SALMON PACKAGES

Take four lengths of cooking foil and four lengths of waxed paper—each approximately 12 inches square—and put one piece of paper with each piece of foil to make a double-thickness parcel with foil on the outside, paper inside. Oil the uppermost side of each piece of paper and place one piece of the salmon on it.

Garnish each piece of salmon with 1 teaspoon of chopped shallots, 1 teaspoon balsamic vinegar, one teaspoon olive oil, ½ teaspoon chopped fresh dill (or a pinch of dried dill), and season with salt and pepper.

Seal the edges of the foil and paper into closed packages: a "butcher's fold" will do nicely.

Green Salad with Dessert Vinaigrette

Food category = Mix With Any (M/A)

SERVES 4

INGREDIENTS

4 ounces snow peas, cleaned
and trimmed
mixed salad greens (e.g.,
romaine, red lettuce, and
green leaf), washed and
dried or spun

5–6 tablespoons Dessert
Vinaigrette (see page 191)
maple syrup, optional

METHOD

In a saucepan, boil 2½ cups lightly salted water, plunge the snow peas
in, and cook for 2 minutes. Drain and plunge into cold water, drain,
and set aside. Leave the snow peas whole if they are small, or cut them
in two diagonally across the middle if they are large. Prepare the salad
greens and place in a large bowl with the snow peas.

Prepare the Dessert Vinaigrette and toss the salad greens and snow
peas until all are evenly coated. Season to taste with salt and pepper.

Arrange the green salad onto four plates, drizzle a few drops of
maple syrup onto each portion if desired, and serve.

·*Avocado with Tomato, Onion, and Basil Salsa*

Food category = Mix With Any (M/A)

SERVES **4**

INGREDIENTS

*10 tablespoons of Basic
    Vinaigrette (see page 190)*
1 pound ripe salad tomatoes
*2 medium sweet onions (red or
    Spanish), finely chopped*
*1 medium green pepper, seeded
    and chopped*

1 cup fresh basil leaves
*sea salt and freshly ground black
    pepper, to taste*
2 ripe avocados, halved

METHOD

Prepare the Basic Vinaigrette, leaving out the honey or sugar.

Prepare the tomatoes by plunging them into boiling water for a few seconds, then drain them, peel off the skin, and remove the cores and seeds. Chop the flesh coarsely and place in a large mixing bowl with the onions, green pepper, and the basil leaves, chopped. (Place the basil leaves in a bowl and snip them with kitchen scissors until they are fine.)

Mix the chopped vegetables with enough vinaigrette to make a thick salsa, season with salt and pepper, and set aside for the flavors to blend.

Peel, slice, and arrange a half avocado onto each of four plates—a fan-shaped display is quite enticing, with the salsa at the base of the fan. Add salsa to each serving, drizzle a little extra vinaigrette or salsa juices over the avocado, season with freshly ground black pepper, and serve.

VARIATION

Replace the freshly ground black pepper with ground chili pepper for a really spicy salsa.

Pasta with Chilies and Mixed Sweet Peppers

Food category = Carbohydrate (C)

SERVES 4

INGREDIENTS

4 large peppers (1 green, 3 of other colors) seeded and thinly sliced lengthwise

2 hot red chili peppers, seeded and finely sliced

4 tablespoons olive oil

2 large cloves garlic, crushed

½ teaspoon dried marjoram

8 ounces marinated black olives, pitted

dried egg-free pasta for four (e.g., penne or fusilli)

1 tablespoon walnut oil

sea salt and freshly ground black pepper

1 tablespoon finely chopped fresh parsley

METHOD

Clean and trim all vegetables and prepare them as required above. Take great care with the chili peppers. Do not touch your eyes until you have washed your hands well after handling hot chili peppers. Trim and prepare them on a paper towel and throw away the trimmings immediately.

Fill a large saucepan with water and bring to a boil—enough for pasta for four. Add a tablespoon of olive oil to the boiling water, add the pasta, and cook until soft but just firm to the bite.

Heat 3 tablespoons of olive oil in a large, heavy-based frying pan and sauté the pepper strips, chili strips, and garlic over moderate heat until the peppers are just softening. Add the marjoram and black olives, stir well, and set aside to keep warm.

Drain the cooked pasta and return to the pan. Gently stir in a tablespoon of walnut oil, a tablespoon chopped parsley, and freshly ground black pepper to taste. Serve the pasta in warm bowls topped with the pepper and chili sauté.

White Wine Ice

Food category = Carbohydrate (C)

SERVES 4

INGREDIENTS

¾ cup granulated sugar
7 fluid ounces cold water
1 tablespoon lemon juice
1 tablespoon lime juice

½ tablespoon clear honey
half bottle of white wine
finely grated lemon and lime
    peel, for garnish

METHOD

In a large, heavy-based saucepan dissolve the sugar in the water and bring to a boil over moderate heat. Remove from heat and allow to cool. Add lemon and lime juices, honey, and wine. Mix well until the honey is dissolved, then transfer to a large bowl or tub for freezing.

Place the bowl in the freezer and freeze the mixture until partially frozen. Ice crystals should be forming around the edges of the bowl.

Remove the bowl from the freezer and beat the mixture until the ice crystals are dispersed. You can do this with a fork or more rapidly in a blender or food processor.

Return the bowl to the freezer and repeat the beating/blending twice more until the mixture is firming up evenly. Allow the Wine Ice to freeze firm.

Place the Wine Ice in the refrigerator about 30 minutes before serving time, to soften. Scoop into cold dessert dishes or robust glasses, garnish with very finely grated lemon and lime peel. Serve.

Day 2 Option A

Creamy Onion Soup
Food category = Mix With Any (M/A)

SERVES 4

INGREDIENTS

1½ pounds onion, finely
  chopped
1 cup diced celery root
1 medium leek, white part only,
  washed and chopped
1 small clove garlic, chopped
  (optional)
olive oil
3½ cups Basic Vegetable
  Stock (see page 194)

sea salt and freshly ground black
  pepper, to taste
½ cup finely sliced onion, for
  garnish
light cream, to taste (up to
  2 tablespoons)
1 teaspoon very finely chopped fresh
  sage, for garnish

METHOD

In a large saucepan, soften all the vegetables in 2 tablespoons of olive oil over low heat, stirring occasionally, until the onions are tender but not browning, about 5–10 minutes.

Add half the vegetable stock and season lightly with salt and freshly ground black pepper (do not use salt if using stock cubes). Bring to a simmer, stirring occasionally, cover, and simmer for 25 minutes.

While simmering, fry the onion slices kept for garnish in a little hot oil until well browned and starting to crisp. Set them aside on paper towels to drain.

Purée the soup in a blender or food processor until smooth. If a very smooth soup is required, pass it through a fine sieve.

Return the soup to the saucepan and keep it warm but not simmering while you adjust the consistency and flavor by adding, to your taste, as much of the remaining stock, salt, and freshly ground black pepper, and light cream as you require.

Serve in warm bowls topped with crispy fried onions and a pinch of finely chopped fresh sage.

VARIATION

A lighter soup can be made by replacing the cream with up to 1¼ cups of skim milk, but this will make it a protein soup, suitable only for use in meals containing proteins and no carbohydrates.

Warm Salad of Mixed Mushrooms
Food category = Mix With Any (M/A)

SERVES 4

INGREDIENTS

½ cup raw walnut kernels
mixed salad greens, your choice
   (e.g., spinach, red lettuce,
   butter lettuce)
1 portion Basic Vinaigrette
   (see page 190)
2 tablespoons olive oil
1 ounce unsalted butter
1 pound mixed mushrooms,
   your choice (e.g., white,
   brown, shiitake, oyster,

chanterelle, cepe),
   wiped clean, trimmed, and
   cut to even sizes
1–2 cloves garlic, finely crushed,
   optional
sea salt and freshly ground black
   pepper, to taste
toasted sesame oil

METHOD

Heat a large, heavy-based pan over a fairly high heat and dry sauté the walnut kernels until evenly colored. Set aside to cool, then remove the skins by rubbing in paper towels and break into large pieces.

Prepare and mix the salad greens in a large bowl. Prepare the dressing.

Heat the olive oil and butter in the heavy-based pan over fairly high heat and sauté the mushrooms and garlic, if used, together for 3–4 minutes, omitting oyster mushrooms, if used. Stir frequently to ensure the mushrooms are evenly sealed and browned, and to avoid the mushrooms seeping water. Dress and toss the salad while cooking the mushrooms.

If oyster mushrooms are used, set the other mushrooms aside on a warm plate, when cooked, and flash-fry the oyster mushrooms separately in a hot pan over high heat for 30–60 seconds. Add the previously cooked mushrooms and stir together for a further 30 seconds. Remove from the heat, stir in the walnut pieces, and season to taste with salt and pepper.

Place salad greens on each of four plates, arrange the mushroom and walnut sauté among the leaves, drizzle 5–6 drops of sesame oil onto each salad, and serve immediately.

Cheese and Walnuts with Crudités

Food category = Protein (P)

SERVES 4

INGREDIENTS

4 ounces cream cheese
3–6 tablespoons finely chopped
   fresh chives
crudités, your choice (see page
   192) (e.g., carrot, red pepper,
   cauliflower, celery, chicory)

freshly ground black pepper, to
   taste
selection of 3 cow's milk cheeses
   (e.g., Stilton, Brie, blue cheese)
walnuts (shelled or whole)

METHOD

In a mixing bowl beat the cream cheese until soft. Add the chives, mix well but gently, and set aside in a cool place.

Prepare your selection of crudités. Select one or two pieces and slice finely for garnish. Arrange four plates: place a scoop of the cream cheese and chive mixture in the center of each plate with a little black pepper sprinkled over. Place a slice of each of the three selected cheeses (serving the cheeses individually means you can control the portions for those who are concerned about their weight) around the edge of each plate. Position a small selection of crudités and a few walnuts in a sunburst arrangement from the cream cheese center-piece. Garnish with a little of the finely sliced crudités. Serve the remaining crudités on a plate for everyone.

VARIATIONS

Instead of mixing the chives into the cream cheese try these delicious alternatives. Do not beat the chives into the cheese, but add them to a herb and spice mixture in which you roll the cheese.

The cream cheese may be shaped into a thin log by rolling it, when cold, on waxed paper sprinkled with crushed black pepper, finely chopped chives and garlic, and a light portion of a favorite fresh herb, such as parsley.

Also, you may wish to finely chop the walnuts and either beat them into the cheese or add them to the coating mixture instead of serving them separately.

To make the coated cheese rolls, stir all the herb and spice ingredients together, spread on the paper, and roll the cream cheese gently back and forth until the roll is completely covered. Chill until ready to serve, then slice into rounds or serve one thin roll per person.

Cauliflower Cheese Soup

Food category = Protein (P)

SERVES 4

INGREDIENTS

1 ounce unsalted butter
1 large onion, finely chopped
3½ cups Basic Vegetable
  Stock (see page 194)
2 medium heads cauliflower, in
  large pieces
sea salt and freshly ground
  black pepper, to taste

4 ounces finely grated
  Swiss cheese
skim milk, to taste
Worcestershire sauce, optional
Tabasco sauce, optional

METHOD

Heat the butter in a large saucepan over low heat and sauté the onion for 5–10 minutes, stirring occasionally, until the onion is soft but not browning.

Add half the vegetable stock and the cauliflower, season lightly with salt and freshly ground black pepper (do not add salt if using stock cubes). Bring to a simmer, cover, and simmer for 20 minutes, until the cauliflower is soft. Test the core of the cauliflower with the point of a sharp knife.

Remove from heat and roughly chop the cauliflower in the pan with a knife.

While still hot, purée until smooth in a blender or food processor with half the remaining stock. If a very smooth soup is required, pass it through a fine sieve.

Return the soup to the saucepan and place over low heat to keep the soup warm but not boiling. Blend in the cheese until the soup is smooth and creamy; a handheld blender does this well.

Adjust the consistency and flavor by adding as much of the remaining stock, salt, freshly ground black pepper, and skim milk as you require.

Serve in warm bowls with a dash of Worcestershire or Tabasco sauce.

Cashews and Stir-fry Vegetables

Food category = Protein (P)

SERVES 4

INGREDIENTS

peanut or sunflower oil for
   stir-frying

6 ounces raw cashew nuts

6 medium carrots, peeled and
   sliced into narrow strips

6 ounces snow peas, trimmed
   and large ones sliced diagonally

4 medium sticks celery, trimmed
  and diagonally sliced (¼ inch wide)

2 medium leeks, cut into ½ inch
   rounds

6 medium zucchini, cut into ¼-inch
   rounds

1 small clove garlic, optional

sea salt and freshly ground black
   pepper, to taste

2 tablespoons Basic Vegetable
  Stock, optional (see page 194)

METHOD

Heat a wok or large saucepan over very high heat; add a tablespoon of oil and immediately add the cashews. Stir-fry the cashews until they have picked up a little color, about 1–2 minutes. Keep them moving and watch carefully or they will scorch. Remove them onto paper towel to drain.

Add another tablespoon of oil to the wok. Add the sliced carrots and the snow peas. Stir for 1 minute, then add the celery, leeks, and zucchini and continue to stir-fry for approximately 5 minutes. Push the vegetables aside and add the garlic to the bottom of the wok. Stir it once then and then add the cashews. Stir the vegetables and cashews over a high heat for 1–2 minutes, adjust to taste with salt and freshly ground black pepper.

Serve immediately into warm bowls with a little of the hot liquid which will have come from the vegetables. If you'd like more liquid with your vegetables, add 1 or 2 tablespoons of vegetable stock before replacing the cooked cashews, cover, and simmer for 1–2 minutes, then proceed as before.

HOW TO PREPARE VEGETABLES FOR STIR-FRY

Clean and trim all the vegetables. Cut the vegetables in a variety of shapes to create texture in the stir-fry; try chunks, dice, matchsticks, flakes, and ribbons, for example. Make the ingredients small enough to cook rapidly but not to become soft and limp. Ideally, a stir-fry should take only 5–7 minutes to cook, so it is important to have all the ingredients prepared in advance. Heat the wok or frying pan over a high heat, then add the oil and immediately add the hard vegetables, such as carrots. Add the softer vegetables in stages and keep stirring. Any sauce may be added finally and allowed to heat through before serving the stir-fry.

Green Salad with Dessert Vinaigrette

Food category = Mix With Any (M/A)

SERVES **4**

INGREDIENTS

*4 ounces green
  beans, cleaned and trimmed*
*mixed salad greens, your
  choice (e.g., romaine, red
  lettuce, green leaf lettuce),
  washed and dried*

*5–6 tablespoons Dessert
  Vinaigrette (see page 191)*
*sea salt and freshly ground black
  pepper, to taste*
maple syrup, optional
ground allspice, optional

METHOD

In a saucepan, boil 2½ cups lightly salted water, plunge the beans in, and boil for 2–3 minutes, drain and plunge into cold water, drain and keep. Leave the beans whole if they are small, or cut them in two diagonally across the middle if they are large.

When ready to serve, toss the salad greens and beans with vinaigrette until all the ingredients are evenly coated. Season to taste with salt and pepper.

Divide and arrange the salad onto four plates, drizzle a few drops of maple syrup onto each serving, if desired, and sprinkle with a pinch of allspice, if used.

Day 2, Option B

Creamy Celery Soup

Food category = Mix With Any (M/A)

SERVES **4**

INGREDIENTS

1 small onion or leek,
  trimmed and finely chopped
1 tablespoon olive oil
6 stalks celery, trimmed
  and coarsely chopped
1 medium celery root, peeled
  and diced

3 cups Basic Vegetable Stock
  (see page 194)
small carton cream
sea salt and white pepper, to taste
2 tablespoons fresh parsley
  finely chopped, for garnish

METHOD

In a large saucepan over medium heat, toss the onion or leek in the olive oil until soft, without browning, about 5–10 minutes.

Add the celery, celery root, and ½ cup of stock, cover, and continue to cook, stirring occasionally until the vegetables have softened, 5–10 minutes.

Add all but a cup of the remaining stock, bring to a simmer, and cook until all the vegetables are completely soft.

Transfer to a processor or blender and purée until smooth, adding cream and extra stock to produce the consistency required.

Return to the pan (through a fine sieve if a smoother soup is desired) and keep warm while adjusting the flavor to taste with salt and white pepper. Serve into warm bowls, each garnished with half a tablespoon of chopped parsley swirled into the soup just before serving.

Steak and Mixed Salad

Food category = Protein (P)

SERVES 4

INGREDIENTS

4 tablespoons finely grated
   fresh ginger root
1 teaspoon tomato paste or purée
1 tablespoon lemon juice
6–7 tablespoons tomato
   sauce
8 ounces green string
   beans, cleaned and trimmed
1 cup fresh basil leaves
   olive oil
24 sweet cherry tomatoes, halved

4 fillet or sirloin steaks, about
   6 ounces per person, trimmed
sea salt and freshly ground black
   pepper, to taste
mixed salad greens, washed and
   dried, your choice (e.g., romaine,
   young spinach, watercress)
approximately 6 fluid ounces Basic
   Vinaigrette (see page 190)

METHOD

Measure the grated ginger into a mixing bowl with the tomato purée, lemon juice, and crushed tomato sauce. Mix well to make a thickish-running sauce and set aside in a cool place.

Plunge the beans into lightly salted boiling water and return to boil for 3–4 minutes, until the beans are just cooked but still firm to the bite. Drain and plunge them into cold water. Set aside when cold.

Put the basil leaves into a food processor or blender and purée while drizzling in olive oil until you have a beautiful, thick, smooth, green basil purée.

Prepare the broiler for the steaks: line the broiler pan with foil and brush the broiler rack with oil. Trim the steaks of all fat, brush with oil, and season lightly with freshly ground black pepper only. Broil the steaks to your preference.

Tear the salad greens into a large bowl, and with your hands gently mix in the green beans. Dress the salad with vinaigrette, tossing well to mix, and lightly cover the ingredients. Place a small serving of salad on each plate and garnish with tomato halves. Place a steak on each plate and draw a circle around it with ginger sauce. Draw another circle overlapping the first, using the basil purée. Serve.

Cheeses with Crudités and Onion Chutney

Food category = Protein (P)

SERVES 4

INGREDIENTS

2 *tablespoons olive oil*
2 *medium red onions, chopped*
4 *tablespoons red wine*
2 *tablespoons wine vinegar (red or white)*
1 *tablespoon balsamic vinegar*
2 *tablespoons orange marmalade or apricot jam*

sea salt and freshly ground black pepper, to taste
crudités, your choice (see page 192) (e.g., lettuce hearts, celery, chicory, fennel)
selection of 3 cow's milk cheeses (e.g. sharp cheddar, Muenster, Edam, extra sharp cheddar)

METHOD

Heat the oil in a heavy-based pan over low heat and sauté the onions, stirring occasionally, until the onions are soft but not browned, about 5 minutes. Add the wine, vinegars, and marmalade, mix well, and simmer uncovered over low heat, stirring occasionally, until reduced to a thick chutney. About 30–45 minutes. Take care not to burn the chutney and only raise the heat to boil off all excess liquid if any remains after 45 minutes. Set aside and, when cool, season with salt and freshly ground black pepper.

This meal looks delightful on a square plate or rectangular platter, such as a sushi tray. Draw a thick line of chutney along the bottom of the plate, then evenly space each of the cheese portions just above the chutney. (Serving the cheeses separately means you can control the portions for those who are concerned about their weight.) Arrange the crudités in columns above each of the cheeses, so that a little space remains between each cheese-and-crudités section.

Herby Green Salad

Food category = Mix With Any (M/A)

SERVES 4

INGREDIENTS

2 dill pickles or
  a half medium cucumber
mixed salad greens, washed and
  dried, your choice (e.g., romaine,
  young spinach, red or green
  leaf lettuce, butter lettuce)
10 tablespoons Basic Vinaigrette
  (see page 190)

sea salt and freshly ground black
  pepper, to taste
lemon juice, to taste
small bunch fresh tarragon, finely
  chopped
small bunch fresh dill weed, finely
  chopped
walnut oil

METHOD

Peel and seed the fresh cucumber or drain the dill pickles, whichever
is to be used. Slice thinly into fine sticks about 2 inches long.

Coarsely tear the salad greens into a large bowl, dress with the vinaigrette, and add salt and pepper and lemon juice to your taste, mixing
gently until all the leaves are lightly flavored. Sprinkle with chopped
tarragon and dill and lightly toss the salad. Arrange the salad on each of
four plates and sprinkle a few drops of walnut oil on each.

Arrange sticks of cucumber or dill pickle on each salad and mill a
little black pepper over. Serve immediately.

Roast Fish with Oven-Cooked Ratatouille

Food category = Protein (P)

SERVES 4

INGREDIENTS

1 medium onion, finely chopped
1 small clove garlic, crushed
2 tablespoons lemon juice
sea salt and freshly ground black
  pepper, to taste
6 tablespoons olive oil
4 pieces firm-fleshed fish
  6 ounces per person (e.g.,
  swordfish, tuna, hake. NB:
  or cod, which have already
  not salmon been used
  on other 1 in 5's)
2 medium or 1 large eggplant,
  sliced lengthwise and
  chopped into ¾-inch dice
1 large clove garlic, crushed,
  optional

2–3 tablespoons tomato
  paste
4 bay leaves, each torn into
  3–4 pieces, optional
1 large red pepper, seeded and
  chopped into ¾ inch widths
1 large yellow pepper, seeded
  and chopped into ¾ inch widths
4 medium zucchini, quartered
  lengthwise and chopped into
  ¾ inch widths
2 16-ounce cans of plum tomatoes,
  drained, juice retained, seeded
  and chopped
2 tablespoons finely chopped
  fresh parsley

METHOD

Heat oven to 400°F.

Place the onion in a mixing bowl with the garlic, lemon juice, a little salt, and freshly ground black pepper and two tablespoons of olive oil. Mix well and leave to stand while you prepare the fish. Arrange the fish in a dish, pour over the onion and garlic marinade, cover, and leave to stand in a cool place.

You'll need two heavy-based pans for the next bit. One with a lid, large enough for all the ratatouille vegetables, to go into the oven. A heavy-based frying pan will do for the other. I use an ovenproof saucepan with a lid that's also a frying pan.

In each of the pans, heat 2 tablespoons of oil over high heat. Divide the peppers and zucchini between the two pans and fry rapidly, tossing or mixing occasionally to stop burning. Add eggplant to each pan and continue cooking. This preliminary cooking is to add flavor and mix the ingredients, so don't worry that the vegetables are only just softened.

Add half of the crushed garlic, about a tablespoon of tomato paste and half of the torn bay leaves to each pan. Put the contents of the two pans together in the larger oven dish, add the chopped plum tomatoes and half the juice. Mix well. Cover the dish and transfer the ratatouille to the oven.

Cook for 45–55 minutes, gently turning and mixing about every 15 minutes or so. Add more tomato juice if the ratatouille appears to be drying out. When ready the vegetables should not be broken up. They should be cooked but still holding their shape. The liquid should be a good, thick tomato sauce.

Remove from the heat and set aside to cool. Ratatouille may be prepared much earlier in the day to allow this cooling and blending of flavors. In this recipe it may be served cold or reheated if preferred, when the fish is ready.

Line a baking tray with foil. Arrange the marinated fish pieces on an oiled rack over the tray. Pour the marinade over the fish and place in the top of the oven. Cook for 8–10 minutes, until just cooked. Check by separating the thickest part of one piece to see if it is cooked through. Serve, sprinkled with chopped parsley, on warm plates with the ratatouille.

TIP

The cooking time for the ratatouille can be varied. Just dice the vegetables to ½ inch for quicker cooking (in this case do not use the pulp from the zucchini or eggplant in the ratatouille—each piece should have some skin). Dice the vegetables to ¾ inch as described above for slower cooking.

Yogurt with Chopped Nuts

Food category = Protein (P)

SERVES **4**

INGREDIENTS

*1 cup (approximately 6 ounces)
  whole, shelled Brazil nuts
approximately 2½ cups
  cow's milk yogurt
½–1 teaspoon vanilla extract
  (or choose vanilla-flavored
  yogurt)*

*pinch ground cinnamon
maple syrup or clear honey*

METHOD

Chop the Brazil nuts to a medium texture in a food processor or coffee grinder. It shouldn't be Brazil nut powder, however.

Beat the yogurt and vanilla extract until smooth. Serve into four chilled dessert bowls or glasses.

Sprinkle each serving with ground cinnamon and chopped Brazil nuts. Drizzle a very small amount of maple syrup or clear honey over each bowl and serve.

Day 3, Option A

Green Salad

Food category = Mix With Any (M/A)

SERVES 4

INGREDIENTS

6 ounces green beans
mixed salad greens, your choice
  (e.g., spinach, romaine, red
  lettuce), washed and dried
10 tablespoons Basic
  Vinaigrette(see page 190),
  made with garlic

lemon juice, to taste
sea salt and freshly ground black
  pepper, to taste
4 ounces marinated green olives
hazelnut oil

METHOD

Wash and trim the green beans, plunge them into lightly salted boiling water for 3–4 minutes until just cooked but firm to the bite. Transfer the beans to cold water. Drain when cold and set aside.

Coarsely tear the salad greens into a large bowl and add the beans. Dress the leaves and beans with the vinaigrette, lemon juice, and salt and pepper to your taste, mixing gently until all the leaves and beans are lightly flavored.

Arrange the green salad onto four plates. Garnish with the green olives and drizzle a few drops of hazelnut oil onto each salad. Serve immediately.

Polenta with Mediterranean Vegetables and Herbed Tomato Sauce

Food category = Carbohydrate (C)

SERVES 4

INGREDIENTS

2 large red peppers, seeded
and sliced top to bottom into
6 pieces

2 large yellow peppers, seeded
and sliced top to bottom into
6 pieces

1 large eggplant, diagonally
sliced into ¼-inch-thick
pieces

8 medium shallots, peeled, leaving
root end intact, and slice
lengthwise into halves

1 bulb garlic, cloves separated
but left unskinned

olive oil

1 large zucchini, diagonally
sliced into ¼-inch-thick
pieces

1 small onion, finely chopped

½ teaspoon dried Provençal herbs

1 16-ounce can
crushed tomatoes

1 tablespoon tomato paste

sea salt and freshly ground black
pepper, to taste

1 cup fresh basil leaves

8 ounces quick-cook polenta

1½ ounces unsalted butter

METHOD

Brush the vegetables and garlic cloves with olive oil and arrange in a
broiler pan. Place under the broiler, turning the vegetables occasionally until they are softened and slightly charred at the edges. Check
frequently, as different vegetables cook at different rates. Remove any
vegetables that are cooked and keep in a warm place under foil. An
alternative way to cook the vegetables is to roast them in an oven at
400°F, turning and checking as for broiling. The vegetables will take
about 30 minutes either way.

Meanwhile, make the sauce. Heat a little oil in a deep, heavy-based
pan over low heat and sauté the onion with the Provençal herbs,

stirring occasionally, until the onion is soft but not browned, about 5–10 minutes. Add the crushed tomatoes and tomato paste. Simmer over low heat, stirring occasionally until reduced to a thick sauce, about 15 minutes. If necessary, heat more strongly to boil off excess water. Season to taste with salt and black pepper. (NB: You can use 16 ounces of fresh, skinned and seeded tomatoes in place of the crushed tomatoes, but I find this sauce simpler and tastier.)

Make some basil purée. Wash the basil leaves, put them into a food processor or blender, and purée while drizzling olive oil on until you have a beautifully thick, green, smooth basil purée.

Make the polenta. Use a heavy non-stick saucepan and pour 8 ounces polenta, a little at a time, into 5 cups of slightly salted boiling water, stirring, then beating continuously over low heat until you have a thick paste. Keep beating the polenta over the heat for 3–4 minutes while it cooks. The polenta will become a single mass, peeling away from the edge of the pan when ready. Now add the butter and beat in vigorously until you have creamy cornmeal polenta.

Reheat the vegetables if necessary, under the broiler. Spoon the polenta onto warm plates, drizzle a streak or two of basil oil over the polenta, top with grilled vegetables and herbed tomato sauce. Serve immediately.

Chocolate Sorbet

Food category = Carbohydrate (C)

SERVES 4

INGREDIENTS

⅓ cup cocoa powder

1¼ cups cold water

4 ounces good-quality plain
chocolate

generous ½ cup granulated sugar

½ tablespoon orange liqueur

2 tablespoons very strong freshly
brewed coffee

METHOD

Simmer the cocoa in the water for 5–10 minutes in a large, heavy-based saucepan over medium heat. While simmering the cocoa, finely grate a little of the chocolate until you have about one heaped tablespoon for garnish.

Break the remaining chocolate into a mixing bowl with the sugar; add the hot cocoa mix and dissolve these ingredients, mixing them well. Allow the mixture to cool.

Add the orange liqueur and the coffee, mix well, then transfer, in the bowl, to the freezer until the mixture is partially frozen. Ice crystals should be forming around the edges of the bowl.

Remove the bowl from the freezer and beat the mixture until the ice crystals are dispersed. You can do this with a fork or more rapidly in a blender or food processor. Return the bowl to the freezer and repeat the beating/blending twice more until the mixture is firming up evenly. Allow the sorbet to freeze firm.

Place the sorbet in the refrigerator about 30 minutes before serving time, to soften. Scoop into cooled dessert dishes or robust glasses and serve sprinkled with the grated chocolate as garnish.

Pumpkin Soup

Food category = Mix With Any (M/A)

SERVES 4

INGREDIENTS

1 tablespoon olive oil
1 small onion, finely chopped
1 pound pumpkin flesh, diced
sea salt and white pepper, to taste
3½ cups Basic Vegetable Stock
   (see page 194)

1–2 tablespoons cream
orange rind, finely grated
freshly grated nutmeg

METHOD

Heat the oil in a large, heavy-based saucepan over low heat and sauté the onion, stirring occasionally, until the onion is soft and clear, about 5–10 minutes.

Add the pumpkin, season with salt and pepper, cover and cook, stirring occasionally, for 10 minutes more.

Add all but a ½ cup of the vegetable stock, bring to a simmer, cover, and cook for 15–20 minutes until the pumpkin is soft and well cooked.

Transfer to a food processor or blender and blend until smooth.

Add and blend in extra stock or water and as much cream as needed to bring to the texture you desire.

Return to the saucepan (through a fine sieve if you require a smoother soup), warm without boiling, and adjust to taste with salt, pepper, and nutmeg.

Serve in warm bowls, garnished with a sprinkle of finely grated orange rind and finely grated nutmeg.

Chicken Kebabs with Ribbon Vegetables and Purée of Celery Root

Food category = Protein (P)

SERVES 4

INGREDIENTS

1 tablespoon fresh tarragon,
  finely chopped or
  1 teaspoon dried
1 tablespoon fresh thyme, finely
  chopped or 1 teaspoon dried
2 tablespoons white wine vinegar
  (or cider vinegar)
1 tablespoon olive oil, for
  marinating
sea salt and freshly ground black
  pepper, to taste
1 pound chicken, mixed white
  and dark meat, trimmed of
  fat and skin, and cut into
  1½-inch pieces.

3½ cups Basic Vegetable Stock
  (see page 194)
2 large celery roots, in 1-inch dice
1 clove garlic, finely chopped
1 tablespoon sesame seeds, optional
unsalted butter
white pepper, to taste
4 large carrots, peeled and shaved
  into ribbons (see page 203)
4 large zucchini, trimmed and shaved
  into ribbons (see page 203)
1 tablespoon lemon juice
2 tablespoons fresh parsley, finely
  chopped

Note: You'll need eight to twelve wooden or bamboo skewers about eight to ten inches long, such as the kind sold in supermarkets for satay. You'll also need a wire rack on which to place skewers when cooking in the oven or broiler.

METHOD

In a bowl, mix the tarragon, thyme, vinegar, and olive oil. Season with a little salt and black pepper and add the chicken pieces. Cover and set aside in a cool place to marinate for at least 30 minutes.

While marinating the chicken, soak the wooden skewers in water. Preheat the oven to 400° F.

Measure two-thirds of the vegetable stock into a large saucepan, add the celery root and garlic, and bring to a boil. Simmer for 15–20 minutes until the celery root is soft. Drain, retaining the liquid separately and keeping the cooked celery root and garlic warm without further cooking until ready to complete the meal.

When ready, push the marinated chicken pieces onto the soaked skewers, arranging white and dark meat evenly. Do not pack the pieces very tightly together. Sprinkle each kebab with sesame seeds, if used, and cook in the oven, on a wire rack over a drip tray, for 12–15 minutes, turning occasionally, until cooked through.

Alternatively, broil or barbecue with high heat for 8–10 minutes, turning occasionally, until cooked through. When cooked, set aside in a warm place to rest for 5 minutes or so before serving.

Purée the celery root in a food processor or mash and pass through a fine sieve. Beat in a teaspoon of the butter with salt and white pepper to taste. Adjust to a stiff purée; add a little of the cooking liquor to moisten, or warm over a low heat, beating continuously, to dry the purée if necessary.

Bring the remaining vegetable stock to a boil in a large saucepan or wok. Toss the carrot ribbons in the stock, cover, and poach for 4–5 minutes until just soft. After 2 minutes add the zucchini ribbons, toss, cover, and poach together for the final 2–3 minutes. Lift the vegetable ribbons from the stock and turn into a bowl, season to taste with lemon juice, salt, and freshly ground black pepper.

Serve the cooked chicken on or off the skewers, on beds of carrot and zucchini ribbons with scoops of celery root purée, scattering a little chopped parsley over.

Green Salad with Dessert Vinaigrette

Food category = Mix With Any (M/A)

SERVES **4**

See page 208 (Day 1 Option B) and page 220 (Day 2 Option B) for variations of your Green Salad with Dessert Vinaigrette. Try topping the salad with a pinch of nutmeg and a drizzle of honey.

Day 3 Option B

Mushroom Soup

Food category = Mix With Any (M/A)

SERVES **4**

See page 196 (Day 1 Option A) for the recipe for your Mushroom Soup.

Roasted Herbed Vegetables with Pine Nuts and Tomatoes

Food category = Protein (P)

SERVES 4

INGREDIENTS

4 medium parsnips, peeled and
  sliced thickly lengthwise
8 medium carrots, peeled and
  sliced thickly lengthwise
1 large bulb fennel, trimmed
  and quartered lengthwise
4 medium raw beets, scrubbed
olive oil
4 large bay leaves, torn
  into quarters

1 bunch fresh rosemary, broken
  into 8 sprigs
sea salt and freshly ground black
  pepper, to taste
8 large ripe tomatoes
  (preferably plum type),
  halved and seeded
2 large heads chicory, trimmed and
  halved lengthwise
½ teaspoon dried marjoram

FOR THE TOMATO SAUCE

1 tablespoon olive oil
1 small onion, finely chopped
1 small clove garlic, crushed
½ teaspoon dried marjoram
1 16-ounce can
  crushed tomatoes

1 tablespoon tomato paste
sea salt and freshly ground black
  pepper, to taste
4 ounces pine nuts
1 cup fresh basil leaves
olive oil
1 cup marinated black olives,
  optional

METHOD

Preheat the oven to 400°F.

Blanch the parsnips, carrots, and fennel for 2–3 minutes in lightly salted boiling water. Lift from the water, drain well, and set aside. Blanch the beets for 5 minutes in the boiling water, drain well, and set aside. Hold the beets with a cloth or fork and carefully trim each, then quarter them and peel the quarters. The beet "bleeds" its color, so wear protective clothing.

Brush all the root vegetables and the fennel with olive oil and arrange in a roasting pan. Scatter with pieces of bay leaf and rosemary. Season with salt and freshly ground black pepper. Roast for 30–40 minutes, turning the vegetables occasionally until they are cooked and well colored.

Meanwhile, brush the tomato and chicory halves with olive oil, arrange in a shallow roasting pan, scatter with dried marjoram, and season lightly with salt and freshly ground black pepper. Place in the top part of the oven and roast for 30 minutes, turning the chicory at least once. The tomatoes and chicory should be slightly charred at the edges and the chicory softening but still firm to the bite. Finish in a broiler prior to serving if desired.

Make the tomato sauce. Heat the oil in a deep, heavy-based pan over a low heat and sauté the onion and garlic with the marjoram, stirring occasionally, until the onion is soft but not browned, about 5–10 minutes. Add the crushed tomatoes and tomato paste. Simmer over low heat, stirring occasionally until reduced to a thick sauce, which should take about 15–20 minutes. If necessary, heat more strongly to boil off excess water. Season to taste with salt and black pepper. (NB: You can use 16 ounces of fresh, skinned, and seeded tomatoes in place of the crushed tomatoes, but I find this sauce simpler and tastier.)

Toast the pine nuts in the broiler. Shake them all the time and keep watching until they just take on a little color. Set them aside.

Make some Basil Purée. Wash the basil leaves, put them into a food processor or blender, and purée while drizzling olive oil on until you have a beautifully thick, green, smooth Basil Purée.

To serve, drizzle a few spoons full of tomato sauce onto four warm plates. Arrange root vegetables, tomato halves, and roast chicory on top, drizzle on a little Basil Purée, scatter grilled pine nuts and black olives over, if desired, and serve immediately.

Green Salad with Dessert Vinaigrette

Food category = Mix With Any (M/A)

SERVES 4

See page 208 (Day 1 Option B) and page 220 (Day 2 Option A) for variations of your Green Salad with Dessert Vinaigrette.

Herby Green Salad

Food category = Mix With Any (M/A)

SERVES 4

INGREDIENTS

*mixed salad greens, your choice
washed and dried, (e.g., red
green leaf lettuce, young
spinach, butter lettuce)
10 tablespoons Basic
Vinaigrette (see page 190)
sea salt and freshly ground
black pepper, to taste*

*lemon juice
small bunch fresh thyme, finely
chopped
¼ cup finely chopped fresh basil
hazelnut oil
1 small green onion, finely chopped,
optional*

METHOD

Mix coarsely torn salad greens in a large bowl, dress the leaves with Basic Vinaigrette, salt and pepper and lemon juice to your taste. Gently mix until all the leaves are lightly coated. Sprinkle on a teaspoon of each of the chopped herbs and lightly toss into the salad. Arrange the salad on each of four plates. Sprinkle a few drops of hazelnut oil on each salad and garnish with a little chopped onion if desired. Serve immediately.

Chicken Breasts Stuffed with Spicy Vegetables on Spinach with Purée of Carrots

Food category = Protein (P)

SERVES 4

INGREDIENTS

unsalted butter at room
   temperature
½ teaspoon medium curry powder
1 shallot, finely chopped
1 medium carrot, finely
   shredded or grated
1 medium zucchini, finely
   shredded or grated
½ teaspoon finely grated fresh
   ginger root
4 skinless and boneless chicken
   breasts (about 6 ounces each)
olive oil

sea salt and freshly ground
   black pepper, to taste
1¼ cups Basic Vegetable Stock
   (see page 194)
1 pound carrots, in 1 inch
   dice
1 pound fresh spinach, washed,
   trimmed
pinch freshly grated nutmeg
2 tablespoons finely chopped fresh
   cilantro, for garnish

METHOD

Preheat the oven to 400°F.

Heat a teaspoon of butter in a heavy-based pan over low heat and sauté the shallot with the curry powder, stirring occasionally until the shallot is soft. Add the grated carrot, zucchini, and ginger and continue to mix and cook together until all the ingredients are soft and the mixture can be used as a fairly dry stuffing. Set aside.

Trim the chicken breasts—do not remove the fillet from the underside—and gently but firmly beat them flatter between sheets of plastic wrap. They need to be about ½ inch thick but not pulverized and breaking up.

Lightly oil four pieces of cooking foil about 15 inches by 12 inches. Season the skinned side of a chicken breast with a little salt and freshly ground black pepper. Place the chicken breast seasoned side down in the middle of the oiled foil and spread about a tablespoon of the vegetable stuffing down the center of the fillet side. Pick up the edge of the foil and roll the breast around the stuffing, tucking one edge of the foil in, so you can make a sausage shape of the foil with the chicken breast rolled inside. Twist the ends of the rolled foil onto the chicken breast to make a package shape. Take care not to overtwist the ends, but the chicken must be sealed in. Remove excess foil from the ends to leave about a 1-inch twist at each end. Take four more pieces of foil about 12 inches square and roll and twist each chicken breast again to give them another foil covering.

Place the foil-wrapped chicken breasts on a baking sheet in the hot oven; cook for 30–35 minutes. When cooked, set aside to rest for at least 5 minutes before serving.

Meanwhile, bring the vegetable stock to a boil in a saucepan. Add the carrots and simmer for 15–20 minutes, until the carrots are soft. Drain, keeping the liquid. Purée the carrots in a food processor or mash and pass through a fine sieve. Beat in a teaspoon of butter, and salt and pepper to taste. Adjust to a stiff purée: add a little of the cooking liquid if too dry, or warm over moderate heat, while beating continuously, to drive off excess moisture if too moist.

Put the spinach in a large saucepan with a teaspoon of unsalted butter and a good pinch of freshly grated nutmeg. Place over medium heat and cook, without added water, tossing occasionally until the leaves are all just softened, about 7 minutes. Drain well.

To serve, arrange about a quarter of the spinach on each of four warm plates. Unwrap the chicken breasts, then slice and arrange a rolled, stuffed chicken breast on each bed of spinach. Place a scoop of carrot purée on each plate and scatter a little chopped cilantro over. Serve immediately.

TIP

Make a butter sauce, if desired, by blending 2–3 ounces of butter in with the cooking liquid from the carrots. Stir over a low heat until you have a smooth sauce.

Yogurt with Chopped Nuts

Food category = Protein (P)

SERVES 4

INGREDIENTS

1 cup (approximately 5 ounces)
  whole shelled raw almonds
approximately 2½ cups
  cow's milk yogurt
1 teaspoon vanilla extract (or
  choose vanilla flavored yogurt)

¼ teaspoon ground cloves
approximately 2 tablespoons maple
  syrup or clear honey

METHOD

Chop the almonds to a medium texture in a food processor or coffee grinder. You don't want almond powder for this, however.

Beat the yogurt with the vanilla extract until smooth.

Serve into four chilled dessert bowls or glasses. Sprinkle with ground cloves and chopped almonds. Drizzle a very small amount of maple syrup or clear honey over each bowl and serve.

Day 4 Option A

Creamy Onion Soup

Food category = Mix With Any (M/A)

SERVES 4

See page 212 (Day 2 Option A) for the recipe for your Creamy Onion Soup.

Potatoes Sicilian-style with Green Salad

Food category = Carbohydrate (C)

SERVES 4

INGREDIENTS

4 tablespoons olive oil

approximately 2 pounds smooth-
    skinned new potatoes,
    scrubbed and halved or
    quartered to about 1-inch dice

10 ounces large green olives
    in brine

6 whole bay leaves, torn into
    halves or quarters

sea salt and freshly ground
    black pepper, to taste

2 16-ounce cans Italian plum
    tomatoes

1 16-ounce can chopped tomatoes

2 tablespoons tomato paste

12 ounces frozen petit pois
    (small peas)

See page 188 for Green Salad
    suggestions

See page 190 for Basic Vinaigrette

METHOD

In a very large, heavy-based, non-stick frying pan, warm the olive oil over medium heat. Add the potatoes, green olives, bay leaves, and plenty of salt and freshly ground black pepper. Mix until all the ingredients are well distributed. Remove from heat.

Empty the cans of Italian plum tomatoes into a bowl. Remove and discard the core ends and seeds, then chop the tomato flesh and add it, with the juice, to the pan with the potatoes. Return the pan to medium heat. Add half of the can of chopped tomatoes and the tomato purée. Mix well and bring to a simmer. Cover and simmer for 25 minutes to allow the tomatoes to reduce to a thick sauce and the potatoes to cook almost through. Stir occasionally.

Add the frozen peas, stir well, and return to the simmer for about five minutes. Test the potatoes are cooked through with the point of a sharp knife. If the sauce needs adjustment, boil off excess rapidly or add a little extra chopped tomatoes. This is a delicious rustic dish and tastes even better if eaten warm rather than hot. When ready, serve the potatoes into individual warm bowls which can then be used for the salad. Any delicious tomato sauce left will then be taken up by the salad.

Mint Ice

Food category = Carbohydrate (C)

SERVES 4

See page 200 (Day 1 Option A) for the recipe for your Mint Ice dessert.

Mushroom Soup

Food category = Mix With Any (M/A)

SERVES 4

See page 196 (Day 1 Option A) for the recipe for your Mushroom Soup.

Quick Roast Pork BBQ-style with Stir-fry Vegetables

Food category = Protein (P)

SERVES 4

INGREDIENTS

1½ pounds pork tenderloin fillet (1 or 2 fillets)

FOR THE BBQ MARINADE

2 tablespoons cider or wine vinegar

2 tablespoons Worcestershire sauce

1 tablespoon clear honey

6 tablespoons tomato ketchup

½ teaspoon Tabasco sauce, optional

1 clove garlic, optional

FOR THE STIR-FRY VEGETABLES

6 medium carrots, peeled and sliced into narrow strips

6 ounces snow peas, trimmed and halved diagonally if large

4 medium sticks celery, trimmed and sliced diagonally to ¼-inch-wide slices

2 medium leeks, cut into ½-inch rounds or ribbons (see page 203)

6 medium zucchini, cut into ½-inch rounds or diagonal slices

1 small clove garlic, crushed, optional

peanut or sunflower oil

2 tablespoons Basic Vegetable Stock, optional (see page 194)

sea salt and freshly ground black pepper, to taste

METHOD

Trim all the fat from the pork fillets and place them in a glass dish. In a small bowl, mix all the marinade ingredients together and pour over the fillets. Cover the dish and set aside for at least 1½ hours. Occasionally turn the pork in the marinade.

Preheat the oven to 440°F. Prepare a shallow roasting pan and wire roasting rack. You'll be roasting the pork at a high temperature to begin with, and the marinade, especially that which drips from the meat, will char a little, so either put an inch of water in the bottom of the pan to prevent smoke, or just line the pan with foil. Brush the wire roasting rack with oil and place in the prepared roasting pan. Put the pork on the wire rack, spoon the marinade over, and roast for 15 minutes. Reduce the heat to 350°F and continue roasting for a further 20–25 minutes (25–30 minutes if the pork is in one piece). When cooked, the pork should be set aside for at least 5 minutes before serving.

Meanwhile, prepare all the vegetables for stir-frying (see page 219). Heat the wok or frying pan over medium to high heat. Add 1–2 tablespoons oil, then add the carrots and snow peas. Stir for 2–3 minutes, then add the celery, leeks, and zucchini and stir-fry a further 2–3 minutes. Push the vegetables aside and add the garlic. Season to taste, stir together, and cook one minute longer.

Serve the vegetables in four warm bowls, topped with thin slices of Quick Roast Pork BBQ-style and some of the hot liquor from the vegetables. If you'd like more liquid with your vegetables, add 1–2 tablespoons of vegetable stock, cover, and simmer for 1–2 minutes, then proceed as before.

TIP

Put the pork in the broiler for a minute or two just before slicing for even more color and char-grill flavor.

VARIATION

For a delicious Chinese flavor to the dish, replace the Worcestershire sauce with black bean sauce, delete the Tabasco, and add 1/2 teaspoon of Chinese five spice powder and a teaspoon of freshly grated ginger. Add bean sprouts and freshly grated ginger to the stir-fry.

Green Salad with Dessert Vinaigrette

Food category = Mix With Any (M/A)

SERVES 4

See page 208 (Day 1 Option B) and page 220 (Day 2 Option A) for variations of your Green Salad with Dessert Vinaigrette.

Day 4 Option B

Bacon and Avocado Salad

Food category = Protein (P)

SERVES 4

INGREDIENTS

8 slices bacon
mixed salad greens of your
    choice (e.g., young
    spinach leaves, lettuce,
    green leaf lettuce),
    washed and dried
lemon juice, to taste

sea salt and freshly ground black
    pepper, to taste
2–3 tablespoons chopped sun-dried
    tomatoes in oil
2 large ripe avocados, peeled and
    diced
walnut oil

METHOD

Broil the bacon on both sides until crisp. Drain on paper towels, then chop the cooked bacon into bite-size pieces.

In a large bowl tear enough mixed salad greens for four people. Dress the leaves with a good squeeze of lemon juice, up to 2 tablespoons of tomato-flavored oil from the sun-dried tomatoes, and add salt and freshly ground black pepper to your taste. Mix gently to coat all the leaves. Gently mix in the avocado pieces.

Arrange the salad on four plates and scatter with pieces of sun-dried tomatoes and crispy bacon. Add a few drops of walnut oil to each salad and serve immediately.

Vegetable Frittata with Oven-Cooked Ratatouille

Food category = Protein (P)

SERVES 4

INGREDIENTS

FOR THE RATATOUILLE

4 tablespoons olive oil

1 large red pepper, seeded and chopped into ¾-inch dice

1 large yellow pepper, seeded and chopped into ¾-inch dice

4 medium zucchini, quartered lengthwise and chopped into ¾-inch dice

2 medium or 1 large eggplant

sliced lengthwise and chopped into ¾-inch dice

1 large clove garlic, crushed

2–3 tablespoons tomato paste

1 teaspoon dried Provençal herbs, optional

2 16-ounce cans plum tomatoes, drained, juice retained, seeded, and chopped

sea salt and freshly ground black pepper, to taste

FOR THE FRITTATA

2 tablespoons olive oil

4 ounces mushrooms, wiped and chopped into ¾-inch dice

1 can or jar artichoke hearts, drained well and quartered

4 ounces fresh spinach, washed and trimmed

sea salt and freshly ground black pepper, to taste

10 medium eggs

METHOD

Heat oven to 400°F.

You'll need two heavy-based pans for the ratatouille. One with a lid, large enough for all the vegetables, to go into the oven. A heavy-based frying pan will do for the other. I use an ovenproof saucepan with a lid that's also a frying pan.

In each of the pans, heat 2 tablespoons of oil over high heat. Divide the peppers and zucchini between the two pans and fry rapidly, tossing or mixing occasionally to stop burning. Add eggplant to each pan and continue cooking. This preliminary cooking is to add flavor and mix the ingredients, so don't worry that the vegetables are only just softened.

Add half of the crushed garlic, about a tablespoon of tomato paste and half of the Provençal herbs to each pan. Put the contents of the two pans together in the larger oven dish, add the chopped plum tomatoes and half the juice. Mix well. Cover the dish and transfer the ratatouille to the oven.

Cook for 45–55 minutes, gently turning and mixing about every 15 minutes or so. Add more tomato juice if the ratatouille appears to be drying out. When ready the vegetables should not be broken up. They should be cooked but still holding their shape. The liquid should be a good, thick tomato sauce.

Remove from the heat and set aside to cool. Ratatouille may be prepared much earlier in the day to allow this cooling and blending of flavors. In this recipe it may be served cold or reheated if preferred, when the frittata is ready. The frittata will take 10–12 minutes.

Heat the oil in a large non-stick frying pan, preferably heavy-based, over medium heat. Add the diced mushrooms and sauté until they are soft and beginning to color. Add the artichokes, and cook for a further 2 minutes. Add the spinach, season with a little salt and plenty of pepper, cover, and cook for a further 3 minutes, stirring occasionally until all the ingredients are well mixed and the spinach is soft. If there is any water left from the spinach, heat the pan with plenty of move-ment of the vegetables to evaporate it, leaving only the vegetables and the oil.

Beat the eggs in a large mixing bowl, pour into the pan, and place over medium heat, rearranging the contents two or three times with a fork to mix the egg and vegetables well. You need the eggs to be setting evenly throughout the mixture without becoming scorched on the bottom. If you try to rush, it won't work. Stop mixing when the eggs are about half set and leave to set firmly without any more disturbance.

When the mixture is almost completely set, place the pan in the broiler to finish. When ready it will be golden brown on the top, the sides will be pulled away from the pan, and the frittata will move as a whole when the pan is given a quick shake. Immediately serve slices of the frittata on warm plates with a portion of ratatouille.

TIP
The cooking time for the ratatouille can be varied. Just dice the vegetables to ½ inch for quicker cooking (in this case do not use the pulp from the zucchini or eggplant in the ratatouille—each piece should have some skin). Dice the vegetables to ¾ inch as described above for slower cooking.

Green Salad with Dessert Vinaigrette

Food category = Mix With Any (M/A)

SERVES **4**

See page 208 (Day 1 Option B) and page 220 (Day 2 Option A) for variations of your Green Salad with Dessert Vinaigrette.

Spinach and Pea Soup

Food category = Mix With Any (M/A)

SERVES **4**

See page 205 (Day 1 Option B) for the recipe for your Spinach and Pea Soup.

Boulangère Potatoes
with Mixed Salad
Food category = Carbohydrate (C)

SERVES 4

INGREDIENTS

2 tablespoons olive oil

3 medium onions, thinly sliced

2 pounds large potatoes,
  peeled and thinly sliced

sea salt and freshly ground black
  pepper, to taste

2 tablespoons capers, optional

½ teaspoon dried Provençal herbs,
  optional

2¼ cups Basic Vegetable
  Stock (see page 194)

1 ounce unsalted butter

1 tablespoon finely chopped fresh
  parsley

FOR THE MIXED SALAD

8 ounces green
  beans, cleaned and trimmed

mixed salad leaves, your choice,
  washed and dried (e.g., green
  leaf, romaine)

1 cup finely sliced fennel

24 sweet cherry tomatoes, halved

1 cup finely sliced red pepper

6 fluid ounces Basic Vinaigrette
  (see page 190)

METHOD FOR THE BOULANGERIE POTATOES

Preheat the oven to 450°F and lightly brush with oil the inside of an ovenproof dish large enough to take all the potato and onion slices.

In a large pan warm the olive oil over medium heat and sauté the onions until they are soft but not colored, about 5–10 minutes. Remove the pan from the heat. Add the potato slices (set aside enough potato slices to cover the top of the dish when arranged, over-lapping a little) and sprinkle with salt (do not add salt if using stock cubes) and plenty of freshly ground black pepper. Mix all the ingredients well. Arrange the mixture in the ovenproof dish, adding a few capers and a sprinkling of dried herbs among the potatoes and onions. Ladle vegetable stock over until it is about three-quarters of the way up the side of the potatoes. You may not need all of the stock. Finish with the slices of potato you kept aside, arranging them to overlap until the top of the dish is covered. Season with freshly ground black pepper and the butter in 6–8 small knobs, evenly spaced on the top of the potato slices.

Cook in the oven for 20 minutes at 450°F, then reduce to 400°F and cook for a further 50–55 minutes. Occasionally press the potatoes down with a spatula to make sure they absorb all of the stock. When cooked, the potatoes should be golden brown on the top and crisp at the edges, and have absorbed all the stock underneath. Test with a sharp knife. Finish off in the broiler for more color if you prefer, then sprinkle with chopped parsley and serve at the table with a large mixed salad.

VARIATIONS
Enjoy a great variety of alternative versions by adding finely chopped sun-dried tomatoes or green peppercorns instead of the capers, and a different mixture of your favorite herbs.

FOR THE MIXED SALAD
Boil plenty of lightly salted water in a pan for the green beans. Plunge the beans into the boiling water and return to the boil for 3–4 minutes until the beans are just cooked but still firm to the bite. Drain and plunge them into cold water.

Tear the salad leaves into a large salad bowl and gently mix in the green beans and fennel. Add the cherry tomato halves and red pepper slices. Dress with plenty of Basic Vinaigrette, tossing well to lightly coat all the ingredients. Serve the salad with the Boulangerie Potatoes.

VARIATIONS
Other delicious additions to this salad are grated celery or carrot, shredded white cabbage, or finely chopped celery.

White Wine Ice

Food category = Carbohydrate (C)

SERVES 4

See page 211 (Day 1 Option B) for the recipe for your White Wine Ice.

Day 5 Option A

Avocado Soup

Food category = Mix With Any (M/A)

SERVES 4

INGREDIENTS

1 tablespoon olive oil
1 small onion, finely chopped
1 small green chili pepper, seeded
  and very finely chopped
1 tablespoon lemon juice
2 ripe avocados

1–2 tablespoons sour cream
3½ cups Basic Vegetable Stock
  (see page 194), prechilled
Tabasco sauce, to taste
sea salt and freshly ground
  black pepper, to taste

FOR GARNISH

2 ripe tomatoes, skinned
  and finely chopped

1 tablespoon fresh cilantro,
  finely chopped

METHOD

In a bowl mix the olive oil, onion, chili, and lemon juice and set aside to chill.

When ready to complete the soup, halve and remove the pits from the avocados, and scoop the flesh into a mixing bowl with the sour cream and mix briefly.

Put the onion and chili mix with the avocado mixture into a processor or blender and add half the chilled stock. Blend until smooth.

Add as much of the remaining stock as you require to make a smooth, creamy soup. Adjust the flavoring with Tabasco sauce (about 10 drops), salt, and freshly ground black pepper.

For the garnish:

Mix the chopped tomatoes with the chopped cilantro and a little salt and black pepper. Serve the soup in individual bowls topped with a tablespoon of chopped tomato and cilantro garnish and with 2–3 ice cubes of Basic Vegetable Stock for extra chill if desired.

PREPARING CHILI PEPPERS

Care is needed when preparing chili peppers because of the irritation their juices can cause to sensitive tissues like the eyes. With a sharp knife split and remove the stalk and seeds of the chili onto a paper towel and immediately discard the trimmings. Chop the chili on fresh paper towels, tip immediately into a small bowl, discard the paper, wash the knife, and wash your hands thoroughly to remove any remaining juices.

Hot and Sour Fish on Ribbon Vegetables

Food category = Protein (P)

SERVES **4**

INGREDIENTS

peanut or sunflower oil

1 tablespoon fresh ginger root, finely shredded

1 small red pepper, seeded and finely sliced

1 small yellow pepper seeded and finely sliced

½ cup Basic Vegetable Stock (see page 194)

2 tablespoons dry sherry or rice wine

1 tablespoon rice vinegar or cider vinegar

1 tablespoon tamari (non-wheat) soy sauce

1 tablespoon chili sauce

2 tablespoons tomato purée

1 teaspoon sugar

1 pound mixed sea bass and monkfish, filleted and cut into slices approximately 2 inches long by ½ inch thick

4 large carrots, peeled and shaved into ribbons (see page 203)

4 large zucchini, trimmed and shaved into ribbons (see page 203)

toasted sesame oil

sea salt and white pepper, to taste

2 tablespoons green onion, finely chopped, for garnish

METHOD

Prepare the hot and sour sauce by heating a tablespoon of oil in a wok or large frying pan until hazy. Stir-fry the ginger for 1–2 minutes, then add and stir-fry the red and yellow pepper slices until just softened. Add the stock, sherry or rice wine, vinegar, soy sauce, chili sauce, tomato purée, and sugar, and bring to a simmer. Set aside to keep warm in a large saucepan.

Season the sliced fish with a little salt and white pepper. Heat 2 tablespoons of oil in a large non-stick frying pan until hazy and carefully fry the fish in small batches, taking care not to allow it to break up. Set aside on paper towels to drain and cool.

When almost ready to serve the meal, bring the sauce back to just simmering and cook for 4–5 minutes while stir-frying the vegetable ribbons.

Heat a tablespoon of oil in a wok over high heat until hazy. Stir-fry the carrot ribbons, stirring frequently, for 2–3 minutes. Add the zucchini ribbons and continue stir-frying for a further 2–3 minutes until just softened. Season with a few drops of sesame oil, salt, and white pepper to taste. Carefully add the cooked fish slices to the simmering hot and sour sauce, cover, and cook for 2–3 minutes without stirring.

Serve the stir-fried vegetable ribbons into warm bowls, top with fish slices and hot and sour sauce, and garnish with chopped green onions.

Green Salad with Dessert Vinaigrette

Food category = Mix With Any (M/A)

SERVES 4

See page 208 (Day 1 Option B) and page 220 (Day 2 Option A) for variations of your Green Salad with Dessert Vinaigrette.

Hummus with Crudités

Food category = Carbohydrate (C)

SERVES **4**

INGREDIENTS

*crudités, your choice (see page
192) (e.g., carrot, cauliflower,
celery, chicory, radishes)
4 ounces black olives
a few pickled green chili
peppers (mild), optional*

*8 ounces prepared hummus from
Greek stores or any good
delicatessen or supermarket
ground paprika*

METHOD

Prepare your selection of crudités and arrange on four plates along
with a few olives and chilis. Divide the hummus into four small bowls,
sprinkle with a little paprika, and serve.

Risotto of Mixed Mushrooms

Food category = Carbohydrate (C)

INGREDIENTS

5 cups Basic Vegetable
  Stock (see page 194)
2 tablespoons olive oil
2 ounces unsalted butter
2 medium onions, finely chopped
1 small clove garlic, crushed
12 ounces mixed mushrooms
  (e.g., 8 ounces white or brown
  mushrooms, 2 ounces each of
  shiitake and oyster
  mushrooms), wiped, trimmed,
  and roughly chopped

8 ounces risotto rice
2 tablespoons dry white wine or
  dry sherry, optional
1 tablespoon sour cream
sea salt and freshly ground black
  pepper, to taste
2 tablespoons finely chopped
  fresh parsley

METHOD

Bring the vegetable stock to a simmer in a saucepan.

Heat the oil and butter in a large, heavy-based frying pan over low to medium heat and sauté the onion and garlic until the onion is soft, about 4–5 minutes. Add the mushrooms and cook for 3–4 minutes, stirring to mix the mushrooms with the onions and garlic.

Add the rice to the mushrooms and onions, and cook for 1–2 minutes more, stirring all the time.

Add the wine if used. Reduce the heat to low and stir continuously for another minute to evaporate the alcohol.

Over the low heat, add the hot stock a ladleful at a time, stirring frequently, making sure each amount has been absorbed before adding more. Continue until all the stock has been absorbed or the rice is ready. This will take 25–30 minutes. When the risotto is cooked, the mixture will be creamy moist and the rice will have a tender but firm texture.

Stir in the sour cream, season with salt and freshly ground black pepper to taste, and add the chopped parsley. Serve immediately in warm bowls.

Mint Ice

Food category = Carbohydrate (C)

SERVES 4

See page 200 (Day 1 Option A) for the recipe for your Mint Ice dessert.

VARIATION
Mix about 2 tablespoons of finely grated good plain chocolate into the mixture the first or second time it is beaten during freezing.

Day 5 Option B

Roast Cod on Shellfish Soup with Herby Green Salad

Food category = Protein (P)

SERVES 4

INGREDIENTS

10 ounces cooked shrimp in
 shells
1¼ cups Basic Vegetable
 Stock (see page 194)
6 tablespoons olive oil
1 medium onion, finely chopped
1 small bulb fennel, finely
 diced, optional
1 small clove garlic, crushed
1 small red chili pepper,
 seeded and finely chopped
¼ teaspoon saffron powder or
 ground turmeric

¼ teaspoon ground paprika
1 14-ounce can chopped plum
 tomatoes
sea salt and freshly ground black
 pepper, to taste
4 pieces cod fillet, skin on (about 6
 ounces per person)
lemon juice
6 ounces cooked and shelled
 mussels

FOR THE SALAD

mixed salad greens, your choice
 (e.g., romaine, butter
 lettuce, green leaf
 lettuce), washed
 and dried
10 tablespoons Basic Vinaigrette
 (see page 190)

½ cucumber, peeled and
 seeded in ½ inch dice
2–3 teaspoons mixed, finely
 chopped fresh herbs (e.g., dill,
 tarragon, and parsley)
capers or chopped dill pickle

METHOD
Preheat the oven to 400°F.

FOR THE SHELLFISH SOUP
Peel the shrimp and set the edible flesh aside in a cool place. Retain the shells. In a saucepan, bring the shrimp shells and vegetable stock to a simmer, cover, and simmer for 10 minutes. Strain and keep the broth, discarding the shells.

Heat 2 tablespoons oil in a medium-size saucepan over low heat and sauté the onion, fennel, and garlic, stirring occasionally until the fennel and onion are soft but not colored, about 5–10 minutes. Add the chili, saffron or turmeric, and the paprika. Cook, stirring together for 2 minutes.

Add the broth from the shrimp shells.

Add the chopped plum tomatoes (if you prefer use fresh, skinned, and seeded plum tomatoes, but I find the canned usually have more flavor). Simmer for 2–3 minutes, season with salt and freshly ground black pepper to taste, then keep the resulting broth hot.

FOR THE HERBY GREEN SALAD
In a large bowl, mix enough coarsely torn salad greens for four. Dress the leaves with Basic Vinaigrette, season with salt and freshly ground black pepper to your taste, and mix gently until all the leaves are lightly coated. Add the cucumber, sprinkle on the chopped herbs, and lightly toss into the salad. Arrange the salad on four side plates. Scatter on a few capers or some chopped dill pickle.

FOR THE COD
Heat 4 tablespoons oil in a heavy non-stick, ovenproof frying pan over moderate heat.

Season the cod on both sides with salt and freshly ground black pepper and a little lemon juice. Fry the cod, skin side down, in the hot oil for 3–4 minutes until crisp and well colored. Turn the fillets over and place the pan in the hot oven for 5–7 minutes until the fish is fully cooked without being dry.

When ready to serve, crisp the skin of the cod again for a minute or so in the broiler while you stir the shrimp and mussels into the hot fish broth. Do not bring back to a simmer or the shellfish will become tough, but they will need a couple of minutes in the broth to warm through.

Serve the shellfish soup immediately into four warm bowls. Top each with a piece of roasted cod. Serve with Herby Green Salad as a side dish.

VARIATIONS

Use any mixture of cooked shellfish in the soup, or make it into a fast and tasty fish stew by deleting the roast cod and including chunks of fresh fish such as cod or haddock just before you add the chopped plum tomatoes in the original recipe, above. Simmer for 4–5 minutes until the fish is just cooked but not broken up. Take care not to stir too much or it will fall apart.

Yogurt with Chopped Nuts

Food category = Protein (P)

SERVES 4

INGREDIENTS

1 cup (approximately 5 ounces) whole raw hazelnuts

approximately 2½ cups sheep's or goat's milk yogurt

¼ teaspoon ground cinnamon, optional

approximately 2 tablespoons maple syrup or clear honey

METHOD

Chop the hazelnuts to a medium texture in a food processor or coffee grinder. Beat the yogurt in a bowl until smooth. Serve into four chilled dessert bowls or glasses. Sprinkle with a pinch of ground cinnamon, then with the chopped hazelnuts. Drizzle a very small amount of maple syrup or clear honey over each bowl and serve.

Mixed Salad with Olives

Food category = Mix With Any (M/A)

SERVES **4**

INGREDIENTS

6 ounces green beans,
   cleaned and trimmed
1 medium cucumber, peeled,
   seeded, and finely sliced
4 ripe salad or beef tomatoes,
   chopped roughly
10 tablespoons Basic
   Vinaigrette (see page 190)

freshly ground black pepper,
   to taste
4 ounces herb-marinated black olives
4 ounces lemon-and-spice-
   marinated green olives
2 teaspoons finely chopped fresh
   cilantro

METHOD

Boil plenty of lightly salted water in a pan. Plunge the beans into the boiling water and return to a boil for 3–4 minutes, until the beans are just cooked but still firm to the bite. Drain and plunge them into cold water. Drain when cold and set aside. Arrange beans, cucumber, and chopped tomato in layered rows on four plates, dress with Basic Vinaigrette, and season with a little freshly ground black pepper. Scatter green and black olives on each salad and garnish with chopped cilantro. Serve.

Lamb Roasted Greek-style with Oven-Cooked Ratatouille

Food category = Protein (P)

SERVES 4

INGREDIENTS

FOR THE RATATOUILLE

4 tablespoons olive oil

1 large red pepper, seeded and chopped into ¾-inch dice

1 large yellow pepper, seeded and chopped into ¾-inch dice

4 medium zucchini, quartered lengthwise and chopped into ¾-inch dice

2 medium or 1 large eggplant, sliced lengthwise and chopped into ¾-inch dice

1 large clove garlic, crushed

2–3 tablespoons tomato paste

8–10 bay leaves, torn into quarters

2 16-ounce cans plum tomatoes, drained, juice retained, seeded, and chopped

FOR THE LAMB

4 small leg or shoulder joints of lamb (each about 24 ounces on the bone) or 2 larger joints about 40 ounces on the bone

lemon juice

olive oil

fresh or dried marjoram, finely chopped if fresh

sea salt and freshly ground black pepper, to taste

2 cloves garlic, finely sliced, optional

fresh rosemary, separated into 12–14 small sprigs

NB: You'll also need three sheets of waxed paper about 12 inches by 15 inches for each small piece or bigger for each of the two larger pieces. Enough to wrap each piece with three layers of paper.

METHOD

You'll need two heavy-based pans for the ratatouille. One with a lid, large enough for all the vegetables, to go into the oven. A heavy-based frying pan will do for the other. I use an ovenproof saucepan with a lid that's also a frying pan.

In each of the pans, heat 2 tablespoons of oil over high heat. Divide the peppers and zucchini between the two pans and fry rapidly, tossing or mixing occasionally to stop burning. Add eggplant to each pan and continue cooking. This preliminary cooking is to add flavor and mix the ingredients, so don't worry that the vegetables are only just softened.

Add half the crushed garlic, about a tablespoon of tomato paste, and half of the torn bay leaves to each pan. Put the contents of the two pans together in the larger oven dish, add the chopped plum tomatoes and half the juice. Mix well. Cover the dish and transfer the ratatouille to the oven.

Cook for 45–55 minutes, gently turning and mixing about every 15 minutes or so. Add more tomato juice if the ratatouille appears to be drying out. When ready the vegetables should not be broken up. They should be cooked but still holding their shape. The liquid should be a good, thick tomato sauce.

Remove from the heat and set aside to cool. Ratatouille may be prepared much earlier in the day to allow this cooling and blending of flavors. In this recipe it may be served cold or reheated if preferred, when the lamb is ready. So make your ratatouille before cooking the lamb, which will take 3½–4 hours to cook, and warm it before serving, if necessary.

FOR THE LAMB

Preheat the oven to 325°F.

Clean, trim, and pat dry each piece of lamb, rub in a squeeze of lemon juice, and brush lightly with olive oil. Sprinkle each with plenty of dried or freshly chopped marjoram, season well with salt and freshly ground black pepper. Cover and set aside.

Cut your sheets of waxed paper. You'll need three pieces for each piece, each big enough to be able to cover it like a well-wrapped package. Wrap each piece as follows. Lay the three sheets of waxed paper one on top of the other on a work surface. Lightly oil the top surface of the top sheet and lay one piece of lamb on it. If using garlic, pierce the lamb in various places and insert slivers of garlic. Lay three to four small sprigs of rosemary around the lamb so it will be well flavored during cooking. Wrap the lamb well in the first sheet of paper. Turn the package over and wrap it in the second sheet of paper; turn it and wrap in the third. You should now have your lamb well enclosed in three layers of paper. You can make the package more secure by tying loosely with string. Lightly oil the outside of the package.

Season and wrap the other joints, and oil the parcels in the same way. Place the joints in a large deep roasting pan. Ideally the wrapped joints should be touching each other. Roast for 3½–4 hours in a moderate oven.

If desired, warm the ratatouille in the oven, with the lamb, for the last 30 minutes or so until ready to serve.

Open the packages carefully and save the juices. The meat will almost fall from the bones, so serve one small piece or half the meat from a larger piece to each person, on warm plates with ratatouille and a little of the cooking juices.

TIP

The cooking time for the ratatouille can be varied. Just dice the vegetables to ½ inch for quicker cooking (in this case do not use the pulp from the zucchini or eggplant in the ratatouille—each piece should have some skin). Dice the vegetables to ¾ inch as described above for slower cooking.

Goat's and Sheep's Cheeses with Crudités

Food category = Protein (P)

SERVES 4

INGREDIENTS

crudités, your choice (see
    page 192) (e.g., celery, chicory,
    lettuce hearts, sweet onions)
a small bunch fresh whole
    chives, as garnish
selection of 3 goat's and
    sheep's milk cheeses (e.g.,

Roquefort, feta, creamy
    chèvre goat's cheese)
½ teaspoon freshly ground black
    pepper, or to taste
sea salt, optional

METHOD

Select one or two pieces of crudité and slice them finely for garnish. Wash the chives and set aside on paper towel to dry.

If you're using the creamy goat's cheese, beat it in a mixing bowl until it is soft, add plenty of freshly ground black pepper and a little salt if desired, and beat well. Set aside for the flavors to blend.

Arrange four plates each with a scoop of the creamed cheese and black pepper mixture, flanked by a serving of the other cheeses. (Serving the cheeses separately means you can control the portions for those who are concerned about their weight.) Place the crudités around the cheeses, garnishing with whole chives and finely sliced crudités.

The Instant Guide to Food Combining

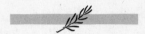

A REVIEW OF THE *LOVE FOOD . . . LOSE WEIGHT* EATING RULES AND ADVICE

Food combining requires you to follow this single golden rule:	Eat your proteins and carbohydrates so they will not be in your stomach at the same time.
Food rotation requires you to follow this single golden rule:	All proteins, carbohydrates, and foods likely to be eaten very often, other than vegetables, salads, and fresh fruits, should be eaten one day only in any five days—1 in 5.
Love Food . . . Lose Weight strongly recommends that you:	Mix fruits only with other fruits, and don't mix melon with anything but other melon.
Special tips:	• *Do* eat simple meals—they are easier to digest. • *Do* make fresh salads, vegetables, and fruits the major part of your diet. • *Do* have only moderate portions of protein, carbohydrate, and fat in each meal.

A REVIEW OF THE *LOVE FOOD . . . LOSE WEIGHT* EATING RULES AND ADVICE

Special tips:	
	• *Do* choose only one protein or carbohydrate for each meal whenever possible.
	• *Do* add only small amounts of fats to carbohydrate meals.
	• Do *not* eat foods marked 1 in 5 in the food directory more than one day in every five.
	• Do *not* drink with meals except wine, champagne, vegetable juice, and black coffee or tea.

FOOD DIRECTORY

Key to the Directory

Protein	P
Carbohydrate	C
Mix With Any	M/A
Fruit	F
Acidifying	Ac
Alkalizing	Al
Neither Ac nor Al	N
1 in 5 food	*
Use sparingly	!

Food	Category	Type	Notes
Abalone	P	Ac	*
Allspice	M/A	Ac	
Almonds	P	Al	*
Anchovies	P	Ac	*
Angelica	M/A	Al	
Arrowroot	C	Al	*
Artichoke	M/A	Al	
Asparagus	M/A	Ac	
Avocado	M/A	Al	
Bacon	P	Ac	*

Food	Category	Type	Notes
Bamboo shoots	M/A	Al	
Barley	C	Ac	*
Basil	M/A	Al	
Barramundi	P	Ac	*
Bass	P	Ac	*
Bay leaves	M/A	Al	
Beans dried (all)	C	Ac	*
Beans green (all)	M/A	Al	
Bean sprouts	M/A	Al	
Beef	P	Ac	*
Beet	M/A	Al	
Biscuits (all)	C	Ac	*
Borage	M/A	Al	
Brazil nuts	P	Al	*
Bread (all)	C	Ac	*
Bream	P	Ac	*
Broccoli	M/A	Al	
Brussels sprouts	M/A	Al	
Buckwheat	C	Ac	*
Bulgur wheat (cracked wheat)	C	Ac	*
Butter (fat)	M/A	N	!
Buttermilk	P	Al	*
Cabbage	M/A	Al	
Capers	M/A	Ac	!
Caraway seeds	P	Al	*
Cardamom	M/A	Ac	!
Carob	P	Ac	*
Carrots	M/A	Al	
Cashew nuts	P	Ac	*
Cauliflower	M/A	Al	
Cayenne (chili)	M/A	Al	!
Celery	M/A	Al	
Celery root	M/A	Al	
Celery salt	M/A	Al	!
Celery seeds	P	Al	*
Cheese (all)	P	Ac	*
Chicken	P	Ac	*
Chickpeas	C	Ac	*
Chicory	M/A	Al	
Chives	M/A	Al	
Chocolate	M/A	Ac	!
Cilantro	M/A	Al	
Cinnamon	M/A	Ac	!
Clams	P	Ac	*

Food	Category	Type	Notes
Cloves	M/A	Ac	
Coconut	P	Ac	*
Cod	P	Ac	*
Coffee (caffeinated)	M/A	Ac	!
Collard greens	M/A	Al	
Comfrey	M/A	Al	
Condiments (all)	M/A		!
Cookies (all)	C	Ac	*
Corn	C	Al	*
Cornstarch	C	Ac	*
Couscous (wheat)	C	Ac	*
Crab	P	Ac	*
Cracked wheat (bulgur)	C	Ac	*
Crayfish	P	Ac	*
Cream	M/A	N	!
Cucumber	M/A	Al	
Cumin	M/A	Ac	!
Dandelion greens	M/A	Al	
Dill	M/A	Al	
Dill seeds	M/A	Al	
Duck	P	Ac	*
Eel	P	Ac	*
Eggplant	M/A	Al	
Eggs (all kinds)	P	Ac	*'
Endive (chicory)	M/A	Al	
Fennel	M/A	Al	
Fennel seeds	M/A	Al	
Fenugreek seeds	M/A	Al	
Fenugreek sprouts	M/A	Al	
Filberts (hazelnuts)	P	Ac	*
Fish (all)	P	Ac	*
Flounder	P	Ac	*
Fruit (all)	F	Al	
Game (all)	P	Ac	*
Garbanzos	C	Ac	*
Garlic	M/A	Al	!
Gelatine	P	Ac	!
Ginger	M/A	Ac	!
Goat (meat and milk)	P	Ac	*
Goose	P	Ac	*

Food	Category	Type	Notes
Gourds (all)	M/A	Al	
Guinea fowl	P	Ac	*
Haddock	P	Ac	*
Hake	P	Ac	*
Halibut	P	Ac	*
Ham	P	Ac	*
Hazelnuts	P	Ac	*
Herring	P	Ac	*
Honey	C	Ac	!
Horseradish	M/A	Ac	!
Ice cream (dairy)	P	Ac	*
Kale (collard greens)	M/A	Al	
Kelp	M/A	Al	
Kohlrabi	M/A	Al	
Lamb	P	Ac	*
Lard (animal fat)	M/A	Ac	!
Leeks	M/A	Al	
Lemon grass	M/A	Al	
Lemon verbena	M/A	Al	
Lentils	C	Ac	*
Lettuce (all kinds)	M/A	Al	
Licorice	M/A	Ac	!
Linseeds	P	Al	*
Lobster	P	Ac	*
Lovage	M/A	Al	
Macadamia nuts	P	Ac	*
Macaroni (non-egg)	C	Ac	*
Mackerel	P	Ac	*
Maple syrup	C	Ac	!
Margarine	M/A	N	!
Marjoram	M/A	Al	
Meat (all)	P	Ac	*
Melons (all)	F	Al	!
Milk (pasteurized)	P	Ac	!
Millet	C	Al	*
Mint	M/A	Al	
Molasses	C	Ac	!
Mullet	P	Ac	*
Mushrooms	M/A	Al	!
Mussels	P	Ac	*

Food	Category	Type	Notes
Mustard	M/A	Ac	!
Nutmeg	M/A	Ac	!
Oats	C	Ac	*
Octopus	P	Ac	*
Oil (all)	M/A	N	!
Okra	M/A	Al	
Olives (marinated)	M/A	Ac	!
Onion	M/A	Al	!
Oregano	M/A	Al	
Oysters	P	Ac	*
Paprika	M/A	Ac	!
Parsley	M/A	Al	
Parsnips	M/A	Al	
Partridge	P	Ac	*
Pasta (non-egg)	C	Ac	*
Pastry	C	Ac	*
Peanuts	C	Ac	*
Pearl barley	C	Ac	*
Peas (dried)	C	Ac	*
Peas (fresh)	M/A	Al	
Pecans	P	Ac	*
Pepper (capsicum, red, yellow, green)	M/A	Al	
Pepper (spice)	M/A	Ac	!
Pheasant	P	Ac	*
Pine nuts	P	Ac	*
Pistachios	P	Ac	*
Poppy seeds	M/A	Al	
Pork	P	Ac	*
Potato	C	Al	*
Poultry (all)	P	Ac	*
Pumpkin	M/A	Al	
Pumpkin seeds	M/A	Al	*
Quail	P	Ac	*
Quince	F	Al	
Rabbit	P	Ac	*
Radicchio	M/A	Al	
Radishes	M/A	Al	
Rice	C	Ac	*
Rosemary	M/A	Al	
Rutabaga	M/A	Al	
Rye	C	Ac	*

Food	Category	Type	Notes
Saffron	M/A	Ac	
Sage	M/A	Al	
Sago	C	Ac	*
Salad greens	M/A	Al	
Salami	P	Ac	*
Salmon	P	Ac	*
Sardines	P	Ac	*
Savory	M/A	Al	
Scallops	P	Ac	*
Sesame seeds	P	Al	*
Shad	P	Ac	*
Shark	P	Ac	*
Shellfish (all)	P	Ac	*
Shrimps	P	Ac	*
Snails	P	Ac	*
Snowpeas	M/A	Al	
Sole	P	Ac	*
Soy (all)	P	Ac	*
Spices (all)	M/A	N/A	!
Spinach	M/A	Al	
Split peas	C	Ac	*
Sprouted seeds	M/A	Al	
Squash	M/A	Al	
Squid	P	Ac	*
Sugars (all)	C	Ac	!
Sugar snap peas	M/A	Al	
Sunflower seeds	P	Al	*
Sweet corn	C	Al	*
Sweet potato	C	Al	*
Swiss chard	M/A	Al	
Swordfish	P	Ac	*
Tapioca	C	Ac	*
Tarragon	M/A	Al	
Thyme	M/A	Al	
Tomato (cooked)	M/A	Ac	!
Tomato (raw)	M/A	Al	
Trout	P	Ac	*
Truffle	M/A	Al	
Tuna	P	Ac	*
Turbot	P	Ac	*
Turkey	P	Ac	!
Turmeric	M/A	Ac	
Turnip	M/A	Al	

Food	Category	Type	Notes
Turnip greens	M/A	Al	
Vanilla	M/A	Al	
Veal	P	Ac	*
Venison	P	Ac	*
Vinegars	M/A	Ac	!
Walnuts	P	Ac	*
Water chestnuts	M/A	Al	
Watercress	M/A	Al	
Wheat (all products)	C	Ac	*
Whiting	P	Ac	*
Yams	C	Al	*
Yam flour	C	Ac	*
Yellow tail	P	Ac	*
Yogurt	P	Al	
Zucchini	M/A	Al	